Obesity

YOUR QUESTIONS ANSWERED

Ian W Campbell
MB ChB MRCGP DRCOG DLORCS
General Practitioner, Park House Medical Centre, Nottingham
Specialist in Weight Management, University Hospital Nottingham
President of National Obesity Forum, UK

David W Haslam
MB BS DGM
General Practitioner, Watton Place Clinic, Watton-on-Stone, Herts
Chair of National Obesity Forum, UK

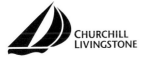

CHURCHILL
LIVINGSTONE

EDINBURGH LONDON NEW YORK OXFORD PHILADELPHIA ST LOUIS SYDNEY TORONTO 2005

CHURCHILL LIVINGSTONE
An imprint of Elsevier Limited

First published 2005

Coventry University

ISBN 0 4330 7453 4

British Library Cataloguing in Publication Data
A catalogue record for this book is available from the British Library

Library of Congress Cataloging in Publication Data
A catalog record for this book is available from the Library of Congress

Notice
Medical knowledge is constantly changing. Standard safety precautions must be followed, but as new research and clinical experience broaden our knowledge, changes in treatment and drug therapy may become necessary or appropriate. Readers are advised to check the most current product information provided by the manufacturer of each drug to be administered to verify the recommended dose, the method and duration of administration, and contraindications. It is the responsibility of the practitioner, relying on experience and knowledge of the patient, to determine dosages and the best treatment for each individual patient. Neither the Publisher nor the authors assume any liability for any injury and/or damage to persons or property arising from this publication.
The Publisher

The
publisher's
policy is to use
**paper manufactured
from sustainable forests**

Printed in China

Contents

Preface

The World Health Organization recognizes obesity as the greatest health threat of the twenty-first century. The rapid rise in prevalence across the world has caught governments and health services by surprise, and the consequences are clearly evident. In the United Kingdom obesity now causes more chronic ill health than smoking, and accounts for more than 5% of national health service expenditure. The cost to individuals is immense with years of ill-health, early retirement, and a reduction in life expectancy of 9 years. However, it is not only adults who are affected: obesity is increasingly a phenomenon of childhood, and carries risks of comorbid disease into adult life. The crisis has prompted some to suggest that we are now producing a generation of children who may be outlived by their parents.

In February 2004, the Wanless Report for the UK government recognized the magnitude of the health crisis caused by obesity. Accepting the role obesity plays in a host of serious comorbid diseases, the report called for a radical change in the way health services should be delivered, demanding a shift in emphasis from a 'national health service which treats disease, to a national health service which focuses on preventing it'. Improving the health of the nation will save the NHS billions of pounds in the years ahead. The concept of disease prevention is not new, but what is unusual, and borne out by research, is the prediction that investing in the prevention and treatment of obesity will actually *save* money, not to mention improve the quality of life of millions.

The authors of this book have worked together for years in the National Obesity Forum UK to identify the optimum way to deliver 'best practice' in weight management in a clinical setting. We have met and discussed the concerns of health professionals across the world, and have found that in Europe, Asia or North America, the same challenges exist. Most health professionals are now convinced by the overwhelming evidence that obesity is a disease in its own right, but are concerned about low levels of professional training and resources, and a lack of local health service or even national governmental support. They are troubled by previous experience of treatment failures and a perception of the inevitability of weight regain.

This book is therefore written for health professionals who would like to provide weight management services, but are unsure how to proceed. It may also prove useful for those not directly involved in weight management but who recognize the need to be well informed, and to be able to identify how obesity impacts on their own clinical domain. It has been written to inform about the compelling argument for the need for weight management; to provide a wealth of background knowledge of obesity, its causes and consequences; and, most importantly, to provide pragmatic advice concerning the initiation and ongoing provision of weight management services in a 'real-life' clinical situation. Drawing on our own clinical experience, and learning from the experience and evidence of others, we believe this book will equip health professionals with the skills to move from simply reacting to disease, to being able to prevent it. It discusses weight management in its broadest sense, and the realistic application of lifestyle change, involvement of commercial interests and self-help strategies, the use of pharmacotherapy, and surgery. It may be read 'from cover to cover' but also provides a bookshelf resource for occasional reference.

Treating obesity in practice is never easy. It requires skill, patience, empathy and determination. The authors hope that by writing this book they are able to help other clinicians agree that the treatment of obesity is both necessary and possible; and although inevitably they will not be able to help everyone, when patients do respond to treatment it can be profoundly beneficial to the patient, and extremely rewarding for the clinician.

We would like to express our gratitude to the Directors and the secretariat of the National Obesity Forum for their steadfast support over the years, and to all those experts in the field, in the UK and internationally – too many to mention – who have guided us and allowed us to benefit from their experience in drawing together the detail required to write this book.

IWC & DH

How to use this book

The *Your Questions Answered* series aims to meet the information needs of GPs and other primary care professionals who care for patients with chronic conditions. It is designed to help them work with patients and their families, providing effective, evidence-based care and management.

The books are in an accessible question and answer format, with detailed contents lists at the beginning of every chapter and a complete index to help find specific information.

ICONS
Icons are used in the book to identify particular types of information:

 highlights important information

 highlights side-effect information.

PATIENT QUESTIONS
At the end of relevant chapters there are sections of frequently asked patient questions, with easy-to-understand answers aimed at the non-medical reader. These questions are also listed at the end of the book.

What is obesity?

1

1.1 How is obesity defined?

There is a consensus between international organizations and world experts that obesity – excess adiposity – is a disease state of epidemic proportions. A disease can be defined as 'a human condition that impairs normal function and implies ill-health'. In 1985, a panel of independent experts convened to discuss the implications of excess adiposity and agreed that the evidence supported the concept of obesity as a disease, and that an excess of body weight of more than 20% predetermined a significant rise in obesity-associated disease.

Although just how to define the disease of obesity remains controversial, what is clear is that the state of excess adiposity – which we call obesity – leads to a significantly increased risk of developing associated comorbid disease.

The storage of triglycerides in an average-weight man and woman, with 15% and 25% adipose tissue, respectively, equates to 10 and 15 kg. The role of body fat mass in a healthy functioning human is becoming increasingly well understood and, in addition to its endocrine influences, the fuel source it creates is necessary for tissue repair during exercise and periods of food deprivation.

Obesity is usually defined using the body mass index (BMI; *see Q 1.4* for the calculation of BMI). Generally speaking, a BMI ≥30 defines a state of obesity and a BMI ≥25 overweight. In an effort to produce alternative diagnostic criteria, researchers have attempted to define obesity by adipocyte cell size, but this has not been shown to be reliable or to have practical applications.

Until recently, the precise measurement of body fat mass was possible only by specialist physicians with access to expensive equipment, and so the concept of body fat mass as a diagnostic tool has not yet been clearly developed or accepted. Recent advances in body fat mass assessment technology are likely to promote more widespread use of this measurement as a diagnostic tool. However, at present, the accepted definition of obesity is a BMI ≥30.

1.2 How common is obesity?

Severe obesity was rare in the first half of the twentieth century and was more commonly associated with the affluent classes, although some unfortunate obese individuals were displayed in 'freak shows' by travelling circuses.

Since the beginning of the twentieth century there has been a linear increase in the average BMI of the population, although in the past 50 years the prevalence of obesity has increased so rapidly that in many developed nations to be overweight is to be in the majority, and to be obese is no longer unusual. In the UK between 1980 and 1997, levels of overweight in men increased from 39 to 62%, and in women from 32 to 53%. In the same time period, obesity in men increased three-fold from 6 to 17%, and in women levels rose from 8 to 20%. Recent UK figures put obesity levels at 22% for men and women. Similar patterns have been observed in the majority of developing nations. In the US current estimates put the prevalence of overweight in adults at 61%, and of obesity at 26%.

What is clear is that levels of obesity have been escalating rapidly and have reached epidemic proportions in many nations and throughout the world in general. If this was solely a cosmetic problem we would have little to fear. However, with the increasing prevalence of overweight and obesity has come a dramatic increase in obesity-related disease. Type 2 diabetes is the most commonly associated health risk and in the UK the current number of around 1.5 million type 2 diabetics is expected to double to 3 million over the next 10 years. We are therefore faced with a disease of epidemic proportions, with hugely significant implications for individuals, health services and national economies.

1.3   How is obesity measured?

The methods of assessment that are most relevant to non-research-based clinicians are BMI, waist circumference and bioimpedance analysis. These three forms of analysis are discussed in detail below.

Many different techniques exist to measure levels of body fat mass. Some of these, including potassium-40 counting and in vivo neutron-activation analysis, are of interest only to scientific researchers because they do not currently have any real practical applications. Others, such as computed tomography (CT) or magnetic resonance image (MRI) scanning, have useful clinical applications. In particular, they offer accurate results and can capture specific organ adiposity levels. However, access is limited to a few specialist centres and these techniques have little relevance to the majority of clinicians at the current time. They do, however, have an added use in helping to calibrate other more accessible methods of fat mass assessment. Of these, hydrometry – using isotope-labelled water – is the most accurate method of assessment in the very obese (>200 kg). Underwater weighing systems have been used for more than 100 years and are cheap to build, although the requirement for a large water tank – big enough for the very overweight – makes them an unlikely piece of equipment in the doctor's office! Dual-energy X-ray absorptiometry (DEXA) scans have proved useful in body composition analysis. They are safe and accurate and, although expensive, their application in several different medical fields makes them an attractive addition to some hospital centres.

Bioimpedance analysis is gaining acceptance as an accurate and inexpensive technique to measure body fat mass, and is usually very acceptable to patients. Other simpler clinical measurements include skinfold thickness and the waist:hip ratio. Selected skinfold thickness provides an estimate of fat distribution, but largely estimates subcutaneous fat. With the development of bioimpedance technology there seems little clinical application for skinfold thickness today. The waist:hip ratio used to be used as an indicator of clinical risk but has been shown to be less accurate than the simpler waist circumference, and so has fallen into disuse.

1.4 What is body mass index?

Traditionally, obesity has been measured using the BMI. The concept of BMI was developed in Europe in the 1800s and was first used to monitor the trends in overweight populations; it was never intended to be used to determine an individual's status as overweight.

Obesity is a disease entity and it is the body fat mass and – more specifically – visceral, or abdominal, fat mass that leads to the destructive effects of insulin resistance (*see Chapter 3*) and the development of associated comorbidities.

The BMI makes no specific measurement of body fat, instead it measures an individual's total weight, relative to their height. Generally speaking, however, by default it provides a crude estimate of an individual's body fat and has therefore come to be accepted as the international 'gold standard' of obesity measurement. The BMI is calculated by taking an individual's weight (in kg) and dividing it by his or her height (in metres squared):

$$BMI = weight (kg)/height (m)^2$$

1.5 What level of body mass index is overweight?

The World Health Organization (WHO) defined the levels of obesity and associated risk of comorbid disease development by BMI in 1997 (*Box 1.1*).

Although no intermediate classification exists between BMI 30 and 40, the risk of comorbid disease development rises sharply. So although a patient with a BMI of 30 and a patient with a BMI of 39 would be perceived as having the same level of risk, in fact the difference would be quite marked.

Above a BMI of 40 the term 'morbid obesity' is used. 'Severe obesity' or 'grade 3 obesity' would perhaps be better because it would be misleading to convey the idea that risk of comorbid disease exists only above a BMI of 40 (*Fig. 1.1*).

BOX 1.1   Levels of obesity and the related risk of comorbid disease

■ Underweight:BMI <18.5 is regarded as being underweight; there is a low risk of comorbid disease
■ Normal weight: BMI between 18.5 and 24.9
■ Overweight (grade 1 obesity): BMI between 25.0 and 29.9; the risk of disease is regarded as mildly increased
■ Obese (grade 2 obesity): BMI of 30 and above is regarded as being obese; the risk of comorbid disease is significantly increased
■ Morbid obesity: BMI ≥40

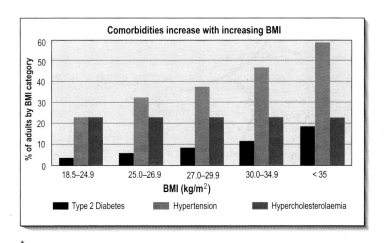

Fig. 1.1 Comorbidities increase with increasing BMI. 'Tested fasting plasma glucose ≥126 mg/dL or self-reported as having responded positively to the question 'Have you ever been told by a doctor that you have diabetes or sugar diabetes?'. Excludes gestational and type 1 diabetes. 'Tested blood pressure ≥140 mmHg systolic or 90 mmHg diastolic or self-reported as having responded positively to the question 'Have you ever been told by a doctor or other health professional that you have hypertension, also called high blood pressure?'. 'Tested total cholesterol of 240 mg/dL or self-reported as having responded positively to the question 'Have you ever been told by a doctor or other health professional that your blood cholesterol level was high?' (from National Center for Health Statistics 2003).

1.6 What are the limitations of the body mass index?

As the name suggests, the BMI measures body mass, not body fat. It is possible for an individual to have a high BMI but a relatively low body fat mass. Typically, this can occur in athletes and very muscular, well-exercised individuals who have developed a high lean muscle mass and a low body fat mass. Even individuals undergoing weight management, particularly those who embrace intense and frequent exercise as part of their programme, may find that although they are losing fat their weight remains the same – because they lose body fat but gain muscle mass their BMI will appear relatively unchanged. The former New Zealand international rugby player Jonah Lomu is a case in point. At his peak, his height was 196 cm, his weight 118 kg, and therefore his BMI was 31, and within the range for obesity. He does, however, have an extremely well-developed muscle mass and his body fat mass is reputed to be only 9%. He is not therefore at any increased risk of comorbid disease. The BMI on this occasion is a misleading measurement.

The WHO range for BMI was developed for the study of white, Caucasian populations. It has become apparent in recent years that some racial groups do not demonstrate the same comorbid disease risk at a given BMI. Chinese and Asian peoples seem to be genetically predisposed to higher comorbid disease with much less body fat. It would seem appropriate to use an alternative model when assessing these patients, and perhaps the threshold for intervention should be changed to a lower BMI level.

1.7 What is waist circumference?

Waist circumference has been recognized as a useful measure of obesity. In 1998, Professor Mike Lean, of Glasgow University, showed that a waist circumference in men of ≥102 cm, and in women ≥88 cm carried the same risk of developing cardiovascular disease as a BMI of 30. This is because waist circumference is a measure of visceral, or abdominal, fat mass – independent of height and muscle mass. It is therefore a very useful indicator of excess body fat and increased health risk.

During a weight-loss programme, a 1-cm reduction in waist equates to a 1-kg body fat loss. Men can find the concept of 'waist loss' particularly appealing, often measuring their success in weight management in terms of their reduction in belt size, rather than weight loss alone.

1.8   How do you measure waist circumference?

> Waist circumference is easily measured using a simple measuring tape. Some are specially designed and carry coloured sections to indicate levels of increased risk. The patient should be standing and relaxed, and shirt or blouse should be raised. The tape is passed around the waist, either by asking the patient to hold one end and the clinician walking around the patient, or by asking the patient to pass the tape around the waist. The tape should be placed laterally at the midpoint between the lowest part of the ribs and the highest point of the iliac crest, and centrally positioned 1 cm below the umbilicus. The patient should have exhaled gently. Waist measurement is most reliable if performed by the same clinician each time. It is easily and quickly performed by the patient at home if a regular review of progress is desired.

1.9   Can children be obese?

Children are very susceptible to the same if not more environmental pressures as adults. The past 30 years have seen a very rapid escalation in the numbers of overweight and obese children. In one UK study, between 1989 and 1998 the prevalence of overweight in inner city children under the age of 5 years increased from 14.7% to 23.6%, and the prevalence of obesity from 5.4% to 9.2%. Similar findings were reported between 1974 and 1994, with levels of overweight in UK children rising from 8–13% in girls. In 1999, 32% of 15-year-olds were reported to be overweight and up to 17% were clinically obese (Reilly & Dorosty, 1999).

Children display the same comorbid disease risk markers as adults. One-third of obese adolescents have at least one additional risk marker and another third have at least two. Once called 'maturity-onset diabetes' we are now seeing type 2 diabetes in teenagers in increasing numbers. Hypertension and dyslipidaemia are common. As many as 75% of obese adolescents go on to become obese adults and carry the same risk of comorbid disease into adulthood.

1.10 How do you measure obesity in children?

The BMI is the gold standard of obesity measurement (*see* Q 1.1 for the calculation of BMI). However, BMI fluctuates throughout childhood and, in isolation, is therefore not directly applicable to the assessment of childhood overweight.

In 1997 the International Obesity Task Force agreed an international standard for BMI centile charts. The panel of experts agreed thresholds that approximated the 85th and 95th centiles. The lower threshold should be regarded as the level at which a child was to be regarded as being overweight, and the higher threshold equated to obesity. These centiles conveniently correspond to BMI levels of 25 and 30, respectively, in 18-year-olds.

In the US, some concern has been raised about the effect that classifying teenagers as 'obese' has on their willingness to engage in weight-loss programmes. Some authors refer to those above the 95th centile as 'overweight' and those between 85 and 94.5 as being 'at risk of overweight'. Semantics? Maybe, but this surely highlights just one of the many special concerns felt by those involved in managing overweight in children.

Waist circumference in children and adolescents has not been shown to fully represent the same level of excess adiposity as in adults and at the current time does not appear to have direct applicability to childhood obesity assessment.

Similarly, body fat mass analysis does not have direct correlation to BMI centiles and is not generally used. However, in seeking to engage some teenagers who are resistant to being weighed and having their BMI calculated, the author has found that many will be intrigued by body fat analysis, perhaps identifying with the technological approach and are attracted by the 'analysis' and read-out that follows.

1.11 Is the obesity epidemic worldwide?

What at first seemed a disease of the developed world has become a worldwide epidemic, affecting all nations and increasingly the developing countries. The US still tops the league with prevalence rates of obesity approaching 30%. Throughout Europe rates have been rising rapidly, even in those countries traditionally viewed as having healthy 'Mediterranean' diets. The UK has the fastest growing rates of obesity in Europe and obesity currently affects 22% of adults. Recently published prevalence rates for adult obesity are: France 7%, Australia 12% and New Zealand 14%.

1.12 Do the developing nations have high levels of obesity?

Nearly all developing nations have rising rates of obesity. In some of these nations the predominant nutritional concerns are of malnutrition, and rightly so. It is a continuing tragedy that in a world that produces more than enough food for the entire population there are still hugely significant numbers dying of starvation and malnutrition every year, while there are others – predominantly in the developed world – who are literally eating themselves to death (*see Fig. 1.2*).

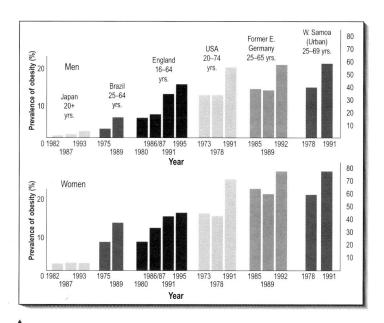

Fig. 1.2 The prevalence of obesity in developing nations (based on data from WHO 1997).

At first glance, obesity levels in many developing countries appear small. Very often data is unavailable or of poor quality. National statistics can mask regional variations and it is often in the cities of developing nations where the greatest problem of obesity is to be found. The pattern of obesity in developing countries mirrors that of Victorian England, when the affluent classes suffered most from the condition.

As Western dietary habits become more accepted the world over, it tends to be the young who abandon traditional dietary habits and indulge in the high-fat, high-sugar foods and drinks that are marketed so aggressively by multinational food manufacturers and retailers. So prevalent are the fast-food outlets that it has been said that the local cost of a McDonalds hamburger is the best indicator of the national economy! Attracted by an image of affluence and 'cool', sales of such foods to teenagers have increased rapidly in many corners of the world.

Nowhere demonstrates this better than South Korea. Fifty years ago, South Korea was a largely rural, agricultural nation. However, the civil war stand-off in 1954 resulted in South Korea depending very heavily on US influence: technological, political and cultural. Over the next 40 years the gross national product rose 17-fold and people began to abandon the countryside and live in the cities. The numbers engaged in physically active traditional farming decreased dramatically and the more sedentary service and manufacturing industries prospered. Over the same period, consumption of the traditional staple diet of cereal began to decrease and dietary intake of fat, particularly animal fat, rose sharply; so too did the level of obesity. Similar patterns, although perhaps less dramatic, can be seen in many developing nations. The result has been an explosion in obesity-related diseases, type 2 diabetes and heart disease.

Another example of increased weight having drastic consequences can be seen in population studies in the Pima Indians. The Pima Indians are descended from prehistoric Mexican people and have lived for 30 000 years in what is now Southern Arizona. They are renowned inheritants of the so-called thrifty gene: a genetic make-up that enables them to survive during times of famine and hardship by efficient storage of energy during times of plenty. The Pima lived by hunting and gathering, and were expert farmers who 'made the desert bloom' by creating complex irrigation systems. They were strong runners and in the 1800s were used as scouts for the US cavalry. However, circumstances changed for the Pima, in particular with the outbreak of the second world war. Many were drafted into military service and others were employed in munitions factories, so their economy was boosted and they fell under the influence of the 'toxic' modern 'Western' environment, becoming more sedentary and buying increasingly unhealthy convenience foods. As a consequence, there is now an appalling problem of obesity and diabetes amongst the Pima, with an obesity rate of over 50%, and they have been labelled as the 'fattest people in the world'. As a consequence, the incidence of diabetes among the Pima Indian population rose to 80% in 1999. Interestingly, in the remote Sierra Madre mountains of Mexico, far from modern 'Western' influences, a tribe of Indians with an identical genetic make-up to the Arizona Pima Indians shows no increase in levels of obesity or diabetes.

Similarly, in Hawaii, diabetes-related mortality is six times that of the general US population and in some aboriginal communities the rate of diabetes is as high as 33%. The plight of the Pima Indians and also the Pacific Islanders is an excellent illustration of the differences in levels of risk between different races. Patients from the Indian subcontinent, for instance, are more at risk from the comorbidities of obesity at a lower BMI, and consequently their chances of suffering from type 2 diabetes are higher, at a lower BMI than their Caucasian counterparts. It has been proposed that a different scale should be used to define overweight and obesity in different cultural groups, and there are proposals that overweight in Asian people should be classed as a BMI of ≥ 23.5.

1.13 Are there any ethnic differences?

The 'gold standard' for measuring obesity is still the BMI. However, research has shown that some racial groups are prone to developing obesity-related disease at a lower level of body fat mass, and hence lower BMI, than the Caucasian population for which the concept of BMI was originated.

It is likely that people of Chinese or Asian ancestry have evolved to carry less total body fat mass, and are therefore genetically unable to cope with the same levels of body fat as Caucasians. The BMI thresholds for defining overweight and obesity have therefore begun to be redefined for individual populations.

Just where to determine the BMI levels for a particular racial group is now a matter for discussion by obesity experts in individual countries but, as a general guide, in Asian and Chinese populations many now regard overweight as a BMI >23 and obesity as a BMI >27. This raises some crucial issues. By traditional BMI measures, many Asian countries were considered to have low levels of obesity. However, because obesity is a disease state and not, ultimately, a measure of body fat, the true levels of obesity in many nations have been re-evaluated at significantly higher levels. These new figures give a better impression of the true numbers at risk of obesity comorbid disease and of the real cost implications of obesity to the health care systems and national economies.

Similarly, waist circumference was developed from a Caucasian population base and, for a true reflection of risk levels in Chinese and Asian populations, it is better to define obesity as a waist circumference of ≥90 cm in men, and ≥80 cm in women.

What causes obesity?

2

2.1 What causes obesity?

At its simplest, obesity is caused by an excess of energy intake over energy expended. The average adult energy requirements are shown in *Box 2.1.*

> Any excess energy intake over and above an individual's daily requirement will result in that energy being stored. Energy is stored as fat, and deposited subcutaneously and viscerally.

This simple 'energy balance equation' is inescapable and an understanding of it must form the basis of any approach to weight management. However, weight regulation appears to be much more complex than a simple problem of energy in versus energy out. Other, powerful, extraneous forces are at work and, to a great extent, an individual's future as a 'fat storer' might be predetermined by genetic inheritance. Some experts estimate that as much as 70% of a predisposition to obesity is genetic. However, those implicated genes might not necessarily convey an *inevitability* of future weight gain. Our genes are switched *on* or switched *off* by environmental influences. In addition to genetic and environmental influences there are neurological and physiological influences, biochemical factors and cultural and socioeconomic issues, all of which could have a bearing on an individual's predisposition and ultimate development of obesity.

Obesity has been recognized and written about for centuries and it is not obesity *per se* but the rapid escalation in prevalence over the past 30 years that is giving rise to growing concern about the health implications of obesity. To understand the best ways to reverse the trend towards obesity, we need to understand its causes.

2.2 How quickly does obesity develop?

Even before birth, there are factors that might influence an individual's future predisposition to obesity. A child who is born at above average weight runs an increased risk of childhood obesity. Breastfed children are less likely to be obese in adult life.

BOX 2.1 Average daily energy requirements

- The average adult male requires approximately 2500 kilocalories per day to maintain his body weight.
- The average adult female requires approximately 2000 calories each day.

As many as 23.6% of preschool children might be overweight and 9.2% clinically obese (Bundred et al 2001). Through adolescence the prevalence rate of obesity increases gradually to a level in excess of 15% in 15-year-old teenagers and, by the time we reach adulthood, at least 21% of the adult British population is clinically obese, with a further 40% being overweight. This gradual increase in BMI through childhood to adulthood suggests that, for the majority, obesity and overweight develop as products of a chronic excessive intake of food calories over that required. In adult life the average adult between the ages of 30 and 50 years old gains 0.5–1.0 kg each year. Within the obese population, the average weight gain is even more, at 1–2 kg per year. Overall we have seen a quadrupling of the rates of obesity in UK adult males, from 6–22% over the past 20 years and it now appears that, as the average BMI of the population increases, the number of people who are overweight is remaining largely the same but the number of people who are obese is increasing significantly.

2.3 What is the energy balance equation?

The balance between energy intake (in the form of calories) and energy output is called the 'energy balance equation'.

To maintain body weight, the number of food calories ingested has to be balanced by the number of calories expended through exercise and resting metabolic rate. The majority of calories expended can be accounted for by the normal physiological energy requirements that enable healthy functioning of physiological systems and tissue repair. This energy expenditure is known as the resting metabolic rate (RMR) and can account for as many as 2000 kilocalories a day in an adult male; the other 500 kilocalories (see Q 2.1) are expended as energy. A continuous intake of excess calories leads to weight gain; a continuous calorific intake deficit leads to weight loss.

2.4 What is a calorie?

The joule (J) is the standard SI unit of energy. A calorie is equal to 4.22 joules. One calorie is equal to the energy required to heat 1 L of water (1 kg) by 1°C, from 14.5 to 15.5°C. One calorie can therefore also be described as one 'kilogram calorie' or one 'kilocalorie' (kcal). The term 'calorie' is used interchangeably with the term 'kilocalorie'.

2.5 How is energy from food used by the body?

Energy gained from food is used by the body in three ways:

- Maintaining the basal metabolic rate: the energy used to keep bodily functions ticking over; the calories burnt off producing the background hum of involuntary vital activity.
- Thermogenesis: energy used processing and digesting the foods that provide the energy, normally around 10%.
- Energy used in performing additional muscular activity, day-to-day tasks and scheduled exercise.

Around 75% of adults get less physical activity than they should (Almond & Newberry 2000). According to one study, 56% of men believed they were sufficiently active to benefit health, whereas in fact only 36% achieved even moderate activity (BNF 1999). Women are just as bad; 52% believed they did enough whereas only 24% actually did. A sedentary individual will burn off 25% of daily energy expenditure on physical activity, the rest going on thermogenesis and basal metabolism. However, a finely honed athlete will use up to 80% of energy expenditure on physical activity.

Only 20% of men and 10% of women have physically active occupations (Allied Dunbar 1992, Waine 2002) and the extra physical activity involved in daily living 50 years ago compared with today is the equivalent of running a marathon per week (National Audit Office 2001). According to the 1999 Health Survey for England, 25% of us are defined as sedentary because we perform less than one 30-min period of moderate exercise per week, and only 25% of women and 33% of men engaged in regular moderate activity. It has actually been demonstrated that an obese child sitting motionless in front of the TV is so immobile and inert that he or she burns off energy at less than the basal metabolic rate.

Not surprisingly, physical activity levels decline with age and are better in ethnic minorities; social class makes very little difference because activity as part of occupation tends to balance leisure exercise (*Fig. 2.1*). These figures help to demonstrate why energy expenditure is so important in weight management.

Because we need less energy nowadays for physical pursuits, the number of calories we consume has actually *reduced* over the years (BNF 1999 15.6a p 123), but it is estimated that the reduction in calories burnt off by physical activity has reduced by the same amount, and overtaken it by 50 calories per day, and that this 50-calorie difference between energy intake and energy expenditure is the reason why we are gaining weight.

2.6 Are we really eating too much?

Obesity can be caused by an excessive calorific intake and also by insufficient energy expenditure. In all probability, the majority of people who are of excessive weight are overweight because of a combination of both factors. Given the rapid escalation in obesity levels, one must draw the

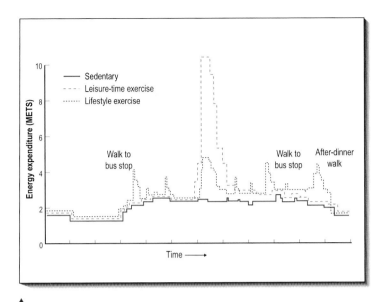

Fig. 2.1 Contrasting patterns of energy expenditure (from Blair et al 1992 with permission from Blackwell Publishing).

conclusion that we are eating in excess of our daily requirement, in other words we have a regular positive energy balance equation. Although this might be because we are eating too much, some studies have suggested that total calorific intake has actually decreased over the past few decades.

However, these earlier studies calculated food intake by monitoring foodstuffs consumed within the home, and failed to count that consumed at work, as take-away food, as sugary drinks and as alcohol. The last 30 years have seen a tremendous increase in the consumption of alcohol, particularly in the developed world, and fast food has become a normal and accepted part of our society. Very often, the high-fat, high-sugar foods provided from take-away outlets are regarded not as a main meal but as a 'snack', even though they might contain as many as 1200 kcal per 'meal' – in other words, half of an adult's daily energy requirements.

Although the total energy consumed remains unclear, what is clear is the increased consumption of empty calories, including sweets, chocolates, potato crisps and biscuits, all of which can be associated with the increase in obesity seen over the past 30 years. High-fat, high-sugar foods are generally inexpensive, very accessible and promoted very heavily. In the 1970s, McDonalds was opening a new outlet somewhere in the world every 3 hours!

2.7 Is good nutrition enough to prevent obesity?

A healthy nutritious diet is crucial for health and weight maintenance. The benefits of a balanced dietary intake, even in the absence of weight loss, can be profound. The harmful effects of excessive intake of saturated fats are becoming clearer. Normally associated with the development of cardiovascular disease, recent studies have also shown an association with the development of carcinoma. One study showed that adult women with a daily fat consumption of 90 g had twice the risk of developing breast cancer as women eating only 40 g saturated fat daily.

The antioxidant qualities of fruit and vegetables, and their low-calorie, high-fibre content, have clear advantages. Highly impressive improvements in markers of type 2 diabetes can be gained from modest weight loss but rapid improvements in overall glycaemic levels can initially be achieved by the introduction of a healthy balanced diet.

2.8 Do social circumstances influence dietary intake?

Many studies have shown clear associations between obesity, poor diet and social deprivation. Children and adults in the lower social economic classes are particularly likely to have a poor-quality diet. Mothers are less likely to breast feed and less likely to provide low-fat, low-sugar, high-fibre foods for their children.

With the decline in the number of local shops, the majority of households buy their food provisions at out-of-town supermarkets. It is very difficult for a family without a car, living some distance from the nearest supermarket, to make healthy food choices. If there is a local shop, it is highly likely that it will not offer much choice of fresh produce, and what it might provide is likely to be of poor quality and high in price. Studies have demonstrated that 20% of teenagers ate no fruit at all. Another study, looking at adult women, showed that only 1 in 5 were eating five portions of fruit and vegetables daily and that these women were much more likely to be in the high social economic groups.

The average British household spends about £3000 a year on food provision and whereas the richer families spend only 11% of their earnings on food, the poorest families spend up to 30% of their income to feed themselves. This 'nutrition gap' appears to be growing wider.

2.9 Are we active enough?

Over the past 50 years the average physical activity levels in adults have decreased sharply. It has been suggested that the average daily energy expenditure of an adult today is between 300 and 500 calories less than it was one generation ago.

An average housewife in the 1950s was so much more active carrying out her normal household tasks, in the absence of automated machinery and personal car transport, that – over and above her equivalent in the year 2000 – she was expending the same energy each week required to run a marathon race! Fifty years ago car ownership was unusual – people walked to work, children walked to school, there was more physical activity within the school curriculum and children tended to play outside for longer.

In today's households, because of reduced prices, it is increasingly common for each bedroom to have a TV, for the household to have more than one car, and for children to have access to a computer games console. We spend many more hours watching TV, and we are surrounded by modern kitchen equipment, which we use to reheat our convenience food.

A comparison of the activity levels of adults in two communities – one built in the 1950s and one in the 1980s was revealing. In the community built in the 1950s, because the majority of households were without private transport, the new houses had been built near shops and schools, areas had been provided for children to play and public transport was essential. In the 1980s community the biggest problem was where to put the two family cars, the houses had been built on the edge of town, away from schools and places of employment. The researchers found that the average adult in the 1950s-built community was taking a 10-minute walk at least twice per day; in the 1980s community it was less than twice a week. Other factors that have led to a decrease in overall physical activity have been a move towards more sedentary employment. Fifty years ago the average adult male was likely to be employed in a factory, in manufacturing or heavy industry. But in today's world he is much more likely to be employed at a computer desk, in a call centre or driving a van or truck. The overall result has been a sharp deterioration in total physical activity.

2.10 What is more important, nutrition or activity?

To produce a negative shift of the energy balance equation to promote weight loss either:

■ less energy has to be consumed

or

■ more energy has to be expended.

Evidence would suggest that the best approach is to combine the two. Those who are physically inactive and are unable to increase their activity levels significantly, perhaps because of physical disability, will struggle to effect long-term weight loss. However, those who merely become more active are usually disappointed by their slow rate of weight loss (perhaps as little as 0.5 kg per month). Increased physical activity promotes the retention of lean muscle mass, which, in itself, is beneficial but that might not lead to a very significant reduction in body fat mass.

An individual can only decrease his or her dietary intake by so much and a daily calorie deficit in excess of 500–600 calories might produce symptoms of nausea, headache and light-headedness. In addition, any decrease in calorific intake over and above this level could result in poorer overall levels of nutrition, with micronutrient loss leading to vitamin and mineral deficiency. It would therefore appear that, for the majority of overweight people, the most sensible approach towards weight loss and producing a negative shift in energy balance equation is to incorporate both decreased dietary intake and increased physical activity.

2.11   Why are some people obese and not others?

A large part of our predisposition to obesity is undoubtedly genetic. After that, our predisposition depends on our interaction with the environment.

We all know that some people, who seem to be inactive, are apparently able to eat whatever they like, in whatever amounts and do not appear to gain weight. Equally, people who have inherited a family history of obesity will spend a lifetime fighting against excessive weight, while appearing to eat very modest amounts.

It was said of Daniel Lambert – the celebrated eighteenth-century 52-stone man – that he '…ate moderately, drank only water, and slept less than most persons'. Despite his 112-inch waistline he '…ate only one meal a day, never snored, never retired before 1 a.m., never slept more than 8 hours and was partial to the female sex'. This apparently non-pathological obesity (although he did die prematurely at 39 years of age) could have been the result of a variety of reasons, but was most likely the result of genetic predisposition.

'Non-exercise activity' might be significant in some of those individuals who appear never to gain weight. Individuals who fidget when sitting will use one-third more energy than if they were totally still. If these individuals stand and fidget, they will use twice as much energy than if they were standing still and 2.5 hours of fidgeting would use up an extra 200 kcal. Such non-exercise activity might influence an individual's total daily energy expenditure.

2.12   Are genes responsible for obesity?

Just to what extent one's genetic make-up influences predisposition to obesity is becoming increasingly clear. The past decade has seen a wealth of new evidence for inherited obesity. Whereas some isolated gene mutations that confer profound obesity on a tiny minority of obese people have been found (e.g. leptin deficiency; leptin is a hormone intimately involved in the regulation of body fat and in appetite control), as many as 250 different genes are currently under investigation for their possible role in the development of obesity in the majority of affected individuals, and as much as 50–80% of predisposition is now attributed to genetic inheritance.

The implications of these findings are immense. Few specialist centres are able to offer regular DNA screening, but DNA investigation in an obese patient with other unusual physical signs might reveal the presence of an underlying genetic cause for the obesity. Although this would be unlikely to lead to any specific treatment possibilities, it could go a long way to helping affected individuals understand their obesity and providing them with a reason for their obesity other than the usual – mistaken – reasons of greed and laziness. It could also, perhaps, ease their guilt about their condition. Increased understanding of genetic influence might lead to future therapeutic opportunities as new drugs could be designed to target specific genetic pathways.

2.13 What evidence is there for genetic influence?

Although much of our understanding of obesity genetics has come from animal studies, particularly on mice, much has also been achieved in human studies – both observational and clinical. Studies of twins have given us a fascinating insight into inherited obesity and have tried to separate the influences on obesity development into heritability, shared environment and non-shared environment:

- Heritability is that amount of adiposity that is directly attributable to genetic variation.
- Shared environment refers to aspects of the environment directly shared, for example between siblings in the same family.
- Non-shared environment refers to that not shared, for example preferential treatment of one particular child within a family.

Adoption studies, examining the levels of adiposity in genetically related but separately raised children, have shown closer correlations between children and their biological parents than with their adoptive parents. Maes et al (1997) estimated that, for women, 65% of the BMI could be attributed to genetics, 8% to the shared environment and 27% to the non-shared environment. Other studies have shown definite genetic variations in both total calorific intake (65% influence) and exercise behaviour (30–62% reported). Samaras et al (1999) reported a study of identical twins that found that a 2-hour per week difference in physical activity was associated with a 1.4-kg difference in total body fat.

2.14 What single gene mutations have been isolated?

The individual practitioner is unlikely to encounter the very rare single gene mutations discovered to date in practice. Mutations of the melanocortin-4 receptor gene (MC4R) have been implicated in some cases and it has been suggested that this is the most common cause of single gene mutation obesity. The pro-opiomelanocortin (POMC) gene was found to have mutated in two children who, like POMC knock-out mice, were characterized by marked obesity and bright red hair. In the 1990s, leptin hormone deficiency was recognized to be associated with rare, but profound, cases of obesity in children. A mutation in the LEP gene has been associated with decreased production of leptin and, in affected individuals, equally profound weight loss has been achieved after leptin supplementation treatment. However, treatment with leptin in unaffected individuals did not give rise to any significant clinical benefit. Many other rare mutations have been detected but their description is beyond the scope of this book. Further details of genetic causes of obesity in children is provided in Chapter 9.

2.15 What is leptin?

Leptin, named after '*leptos*' the Greek word for 'thin', is a hormone secreted by adipose tissue, whose function is to send a message to the hypothalamus to tell us to stop eating when satiated. There are incredibly rare instances of total leptin deficiency; three Turkish cousins were discovered to have this genetic condition, which resulted in voracious appetites, no feeling of fullness, no signal to stop eating and, not surprisingly, morbid obesity. Leptin injections enabled them to lose massive amounts of weight and gave hope to obese people everywhere. However, the results of research on leptin have been disappointing and no breakthrough has occurred in the fight against obesity. Although leptin tells us to stop eating, obese people usually have a *raised* leptin level. A study by Considine et al (1996) showed that obese people have an average of four times the amount of leptin than that of non-obese individuals, and that a reduction in weight of 10% reduced leptin levels by 55%. Artificially increasing leptin levels, therefore, has no benefit for obese patients, as was originally hoped. Theories – including the concept of leptin resistance – were developed to explain why a hormone that should cause thinness was actually present in higher quantities in obese people. It seems likely that there is resistance to leptin and insulin at the blood–brain barrier and that abnormalities in certain neuropeptides are responsible for the condition. The transmitters serotonin and noradrenaline (on which the drug sibutramine acts; *see Chapter 7*) are involved in the catabolic processes at this level. Leptin also activates the sympathetic nervous system, and thereby has a role in blood pressure regulation and other functions.

2.16 What is resistin?

Resistin is a peptide hormone secreted by white fat cells. It was discovered in 2001 and named after *resist*ance to *in*sulin. It was initially thought to represent the link between obesity and type 2 diabetes because, in animal studies, it seemed to enable tissues to resist the effects of insulin (Steppan et al 2001). However, more recent studies in humans have shown no difference in resistin expression between normal, insulin-resistant subjects or people with type 2 diabetes, although some genetic studies show a positive link between obesity, insulin resistance and resistin. It is safe to say that although resistin might have an important role in obesity and insulin resistance, so far we don't know exactly what this is (Ukkola 2002).

2.17 What is adiponectin?

Adiponectin is a protein derived exclusively from adipose tissue. It seems to have protective metabolic and anti-inflammatory properties, and reduces inflammatory changes in the cardiovascular system that lead to heart disease. Plasma adiponectin levels are decreased in obesity, insulin resistance, type 2 diabetes and dyslipidaemia, and are particularly low in patients with coronary artery disease. This seems to be a link between obesity and its most important comorbidities, and another important component of the metabolic syndrome (*see Chapter 3*). Adiponectin levels can be increased by weight loss and the protein is seen in greater levels when insulin sensitivity is increased by, for example, thiazolidinediones (glitazones) (Engeli et al 2003, available: http://www.diabetes.diabetesjournals.org).

2.18 What are cytokines?

Increased levels of obesity are associated with increased plasma levels of cytokines (inflammatory factors) such as interleukins (e.g. IL-6), C-reactive protein (CRP), tumour necrosis factor (TNF) and insulin-like growth factor-1 (IGF-1). These cytokines are produced by adipose tissue and are responsible for inflammatory changes in the cardiovascular and other systems. This led to the concept of the 'adipovascular' axis, which is thought to contribute to the increase in cardiovascular events in obese subjects (Engeli et al 2003).

Omentin is a recently discovered protein secreted by the omental adipose tissue that appears, like adiponectin, to increase insulin sensitivity and stimulate glucose uptake (Yang et al 2003).

Many other proteins are in various stages of research, including ghrelin, pancreatic peptide YY, neuropeptide Y and glucagon-like peptides 1 and 2, all of which can be considered as energy regulators. These, and the many more molecules that will doubtless be discovered, will be either discarded or hailed as the next great hope in obesity management in the years to come.

2.19 How significant is environmental influence?

Environmental factors are absolutely pivotal to our understanding of the causes of obesity. Despite the very significant influence of genetic inheritance, the gene pool within Europe has not changed significantly over the past 1000 years. The obesity epidemic is a modern phenomenon – in particular of the past 20 years – and is much more likely to represent changes in the environment. If we consider that we evolved genetically to be able to accumulate and store fat in times of plenty, so that we could survive during times of need, those of us who have survived are therefore descendants of those 'fat storers'. It is therefore understandable that we should be able to accumulate body fat mass from an historical, survival point of view. The problem is that we now rarely experience times of need, and our ability to consume and absorb energy as fat is no longer so important. As a result, we are rapidly growing fatter and suffering the consequences of comorbid disease. The current obesity epidemic should therefore be regarded as a *normal reaction to an abnormal environment*. Not only has the environment been very influential in creating our obesogenic lifestyles, it is also where we must look to effect long-term preventive policies and treatment strategies.

2.20 Can we escape environmental influence?

Environmental pressures encouraging us to eat are very powerful. To avoid food altogether is impossible. It is easy to eat. It is comfortable, satisfying and relatively inexpensive. We are subject to very strong physiological signals that make us want to eat and very weak signals to stop. Hunger makes us feel unwell, sometimes irritable, and food is often available 24 hours a day. We eat when we are happy, we eat when we are sad and we have adopted social and celebratory habits that incorporate excessive eating and drinking. We associate an ability to eat well with health, affluence and social status.

Simultaneously, our society has worked hard over generations to make life easier and physical activity less necessary. To become more active is not easy. It requires effort and can be uncomfortable and time consuming. In past generations, large-scale workforces were paid for their physical activity but in today's society, where work is much more sedentary, we have to pay to be more active by joining gyms and playing formal sports. After a long day at the office or in the classroom, and with other tasks to be done at home, it requires a great deal of motivation to expend more energy and take ourselves out of the comfort zone.

There is no clear strategy for changing the environment. Some have suggested fat taxes on food or even tax rebates for physical activity. Some have suggested statutory changes to prevent the promotion of energy rich foods and fizzy drinks. For the vast majority of people, avoiding obesity, or achieving meaningful weight loss in those who are already obese, is extremely difficult. We ask patients to go against their physiological instincts to eat when food is available and to rest when physical activity is not required.

Changing the environment to one that encourages a more healthy lifestyle would require measures to not only educate but also to facilitate individuals to take steps to override their physiological drives. However, according to the National Weight Control Registry (NWCR) in the US, of those who are successful in losing weight, only 9% have been able to maintain their weight loss without regular physical activity and only rarely does an individual achieve long-term weight loss maintenance without significant amounts of physical activity.

It might be that the most significant impact that can be made on the obesogenic environment is on physical activity, and that increasing activity is what we should aspire to and where our initial efforts should be concentrated. For individuals who are obese, treatment strategies must include lifestyle advice and the use of appropriate medical therapies. On a preventive level, and taking a global approach to weight management and disease prevention, we must work towards changing the environment and developing an increased understanding of how to facilitate weight management within that environment.

2.21 Isn't it a matter of will power?

For centuries obese people have been subject to teasing, ridicule and social prejudice. They are usually assumed to be greedy and lazy, and to lack any self control. These beliefs are only compounded when obese individuals attempt to lose weight but are unable to reduce their calorific intake and increase their energy expenditure sufficiently to effect long-term weight loss. Current research does not support this view of obesity, however, and it is already acknowledged that as much as 70% of our predisposition to obesity is genetic. Thereafter we are subject to the very powerful influences of the obesogenic environment – forces that can be sometimes impossible to overcome. Clearly, lifestyle change incorporating changes in dietary intake and physical activity levels, together with behavioural modification, are crucial for anyone embarking on a weight-loss programme but experienced clinicians will always be aware of some patients whose best efforts have been evident but who have not been able to effect meaningful weight loss.

To develop better treatment strategies we need to move away from a blame culture, and to offer support and education to patients rather than criticism; understanding instead of castigation. The physiological mechanisms involved in weight regulation are poorly understood but improved understanding of the causes of obesity does not negate the responsibilities of obese individuals to try to control their lifestyle habits. Will power is difficult to define. You can have it one day and not the next. Weight management is certainly about more than self-will.

2.22 What can be done to encourage improved nutrition?

Education is essential and must cover all aspects of society. The media and the advertising industry are powerful players in today's society and could exert a very positive influence if they chose to.

Within the school system steps are already underway – some by the authorities, some charitable – to provide balanced nutritional advice in schools. An enthused child can carry good habits through to adult life and can even act as a catalyst for the benefit of parents and siblings on the way. Education delivered by medical practitioners in the form of personal advice, information sheets or books, can inform and educate concerned patients. However, after education, comes facilitation and measures to improve availability of cheap and accessible, good quality foods is essential if we are to address the problem of obesity with individuals and in our community.

Much could also be done to prevent adverse influences – on both children and adults – through restrictions on food advertising and by regulating the content of popular ready-made foods. The concern of governments throughout Europe, and indeed worldwide, has led to a greater priority being given both to providing healthy food at schools and to minimizing the opportunity for children to consume unhealthy foods at school. Some schools in the US receive significant financial incentives to stock and indeed promote sugary soft drinks and high-fat food to children. Such sponsorship – by pizza manufacturers and burger outlets – is rare in Europe and needs to be guarded against. The argument that such sponsorship is about promoting choice and brand loyalty is a weak one. The time has come for us to put the needs of our children before the interests of big business.

2.23 What can be done to improve activity levels?

See Q 6.30

2.24 Is prevention more important than treatment?

Few would disagree that prevention is better than a cure. Medically, economically, psychologically and socially, preventing obesity at national or individual level must be preferable to treatment. However, weight management as a medical intervention must be made available to obese individuals, when appropriate, to support their weight-management attempts. If it is not, we fail in our obligations to our patients and miss out on the undoubted benefits of medically supported, moderate weight loss. If the conditions that cause obesity can be improved, and if we can inform, educate and facilitate the introduction of better nutrition and activity levels on a national scale, the health and economic benefits would be profound. Significant environmental change requires the will and support of government and national institutions, including the education, health and medical professions. It will also require cooperation with the food industry, the advertising industry and all individual members of society, who have a personal responsibility to take steps to promote their own well-being. Clearly this is not the situation at the current time and much needs to be done to persuade national government to take stringent measures in order to reverse the trend towards obesity.

2.25   Should we legislate against the food industry?

Food manufacturers are already obliged to put nutritional information labels on any foods that claim to offer nutritional benefits. Despite this, the number of food items carrying such information is still very low, and what information is provided is often misleading and almost always inadequate. Any further legislative change within Europe will take time, as a consensus needs to be reached within the European Union before any laws can be passed. It is possible that the food industry will be allowed to continue to self-regulate, although its record to date has not been inspiring. A lawsuit alleging food from McDonalds restaurants was responsible for making people obese was thrown out of a US court in February 2003. The first legal action of its kind against a fast-food retailer, it was claimed that McDonalds and two of its restaurants failed to disclose, clearly and conspicuously, the ingredients and effects of its food – much of which is high in fat, salt, sugar and cholesterol. The judge ruled that food suppliers, or the law, could not be held to account for a customer's voluntary excesses, and the issue as to how much responsibility food manufacturers *do* have remains unclear. In July 2003, Kraft Foods, concerned about the possibility of legal action, announced health-driven reductions in the portion size, fat, sugar and salt content of some of its major brands. In the UK, McDonalds have announced decreased portion sizes from December 2004.

2.26   Should food advertising to children be banned?

There are campaigns in many countries to legislate against the advertising of high-fat, high-sugar foods to children. The UK campaign group, Sustain, estimates that more than 80% of advertising during children's peak TV viewing hours is for high-fat, high-sugar foods.

Although food advertising would seem to contribute to the increased trend towards consumption of such foods by children, there is little evidence to prove the point and any attempts to legislate against such advertising are likely to run into stiff resistance. There is little governmental will to seek change and the food manufacturing industry is a very powerful lobby in the UK, and far more so in The US.

However, some changes have been brought about through appropriate campaigns. For example, many UK supermarkets no longer stock children's sweets at the check-out, accepting that this applies undue pressure on parents to purchase. In Sweden, advertising to children under age 12 was banned completely in an effort to reduce the potential for the food industry, among others, to exploit easily influenced young minds. Such radical controlling measures almost certainly make a positive contribution to the campaign to reduce the ability of the commercial world to make even more money on the back of our children's health. However, in the opinion of the author, we would be better to exert our influence upon the food industry in a spirit of constructive cooperation, seeking to work with, rather than against it, to develop healthier choices, better provision of affordable fruit and vegetables and low-fat, low-sugar foods in small corner shops as well as in larger retailers.

2.27 What is a fat tax?

The concept of a fat tax has been put forward in several countries. The principle is that as fat is so clearly implicated in the development of overweight, any foods that carry high levels of fat should be subject to extra taxation to discourage their manufacture and purchase. The protagonists of the fat tax propose that any fiscal gains from such a tax be used to finance improved provision of healthy food choices in poorer areas. The opponents of the argument point to the fact that the people who are most likely to incur this fat tax – the obese – are more likely to be in the lower socioeconomic groups and that the fat tax is therefore a proposal to further tax the poorer members of society. In addition to the complex logistics that would be required to administer the tax, it is highly likely that the food industry would be able to circumvent the tax in due course. In any case, it is unlikely that a few pennies added to the cost of a hamburger would have any significant impact on the development of obesity at a national level.

Other proposals have included tax rebates for people who are engaging in formal sporting activity, for example a partial rebate on their gym subscriptions. However, there is no evidence to support the concept that such tax advantages would encourage increased physical activity and the inverse argument to that for the fat tax applies here – those most likely to benefit from such a tax rebate would be those who are already high earners and already able to afford gym membership. The logistics of such a proposal would be highly likely to negate any advantage.

PATIENT QUESTIONS

2.28 How and why does obesity affect my health?

Obesity affects health in a number of ways. The extra weight means additional strain on the knees and hips, leading to arthritis; extra work for the heart to pump blood around the excess tissue and more stress on the lungs and airways causing breathlessness. But there is a more sinister mechanism by which obesity causes ill health and death: the fat stored around the waist and inside the abdomen produces a large variety of chemicals and hormones called inflammatory factors, which cause havoc in the organs in the rest of the body. They lead to raised levels of cholesterol and fats, causing heart disease and strokes, they stimulate the kidneys to cause high blood pressure, they have the same effect as alcohol on the liver and they can also lead to around 20 different causes of cancer. The only way of preventing the damage done by these chemicals is by losing weight.

The physical effects of obesity

3

3.1 What is the significance of abdominal obesity?

Abdominal obesity is known to be associated with far greater risk of comorbidities than gluteal or peripheral obesity. This difference in fat distribution has led to the description of people with abdominal obesity as 'apples' and those with gluteal obesity 'pears'; alternatively known as android or gynoid obesity, respectively. In the nineteenth century no great significance was attached to abdominal obesity. It was a relatively rare occurrence associated with well-off higher social classes, although some authors were beginning to get an inkling of its importance:

A large number of people, while of seemly proportions in other respects, grow an abdomen that is exceedingly ugly and becomes in time a great inconvenience. This is because, while the general activity of the person is considerable, their abdomen is kept free from muscular action. A protruding abdomen is patted and petted as a kind of symbol of health, when, in fact, it is sometimes, if not often, a threatening sign. It is at least a prophecy of too much fat, and as such should be looked at askance. (Checkley 1892)

It is now clear that visceral obesity is of the greatest significance. Visceral obesity is adipose tissue situated within the abdomen, around the omentum of the bowel. It shares its blood supply with the omentum and secretes directly into the portal circulation. The amount of visceral fat is proportional to the waist circumference. In other words, measuring the waist not only gives an idea of subcutaneous fat around the belly but, more importantly, the amount of adipose tissue within the abdominal cavity.

3.2 What is the function of visceral fat?

Far from merely being an 'ugly inconvenience' as was once thought, adipose tissue – especially visceral fat – is now considered to be a highly active endocrine organ. It produces and secretes hormones into the portal circulation. It also releases free fatty acids, the products of lipolysis, and inflammatory substances called cytokines, which circulate in the blood and cause havoc in their target organs. Many of these substances are still in the early stages of discovery and research but others are known to be responsible for inflammatory and malignant changes in organs such as the colon and kidney.

3.3 What are the main diseases associated with obesity and overweight?

Physiological and biochemical mechanisms associated with obesity affect every system of the body. Obesity is closely associated with a variety of comorbidities that can occur alone or concomitantly. These include type 2 diabetes, dyslipidaemia, cardiovascular disease, hypertension, stroke, liver disease, respiratory disorders, gout and osteoarthritis, as well as up to 20 types of cancer. Statistics from the National Center for Health Statistics Third National Health and Nutrition Examination Survey reveal that 65% of overweight or obese adults (BMI ≥ 27) have at least one of these chronic diseases, and that 27% have two or more. Furthermore, the impact of these comorbid conditions grows as individuals gain weight.

OBESITY IN WOMEN

3.4 What is polycystic ovary syndrome (Stein-Leventhal syndrome)?

Polycystic ovary syndrome (PCOS) is a condition in which excess androgen secretion leads to the formation of a number of follicular cysts within the ovary. These are detectable on ultrasound examination. The ovaries might be enlarged, with thickened capsules, or normal sized. The presenting features vary but may include amenorrhoea, infertility, hirsutism, obesity (although patients may be of normal weight) and irregular, profuse menstrual bleeding. The hormonal findings usually demonstrate raised levels of luteinizing hormone (LH), a constant, low-to-normal level of follicle-stimulating hormone (FSH) and high levels of circulating androgens. Complications can arise from high unopposed oestrogen levels, including endometrial hyperplasia and menorrhagia, and rarely, endometrial carcinoma.

3.5 What is the treatment for PCOS?

Treatment is often aimed at reducing these risks by giving oral progestogens, or oral contraceptives, once an endometrial biopsy has been taken to eliminate the risk of endometrial carcinoma. Alternatively, cyproterone acetate, an antiandrogen and progestational agent, can be used to control hirsutism, along with a cyclical oestrogen to induce withdrawal bleeds.

 The most distressing complication is often reduced fertility or infertility, which can be treated in specialist clinics with drugs such as clomiphene to induce ovulation. An alternative is spironolactone, which is a diuretic and androgen inhibitor.

3.6 What is the connection between PCOS and obesity?

The high circulating levels of insulin found in obese women with the metabolic syndrome (see Chapter 6) stimulate the ovaries to secrete excess levels of testosterone, leading to hirsutism and other androgenic effects. Like oestrogens, androgens are fat soluble and so are absorbed into the adipose tissue until tissue androgen levels are in a state of dynamic equilibrium with levels in the blood. As well as acting as a store for steroid sex hormones, the adipose tissue also changes androgens to oestrogens, a process known as peripheral conversion. The resulting excess oestrogen level interferes with the feedback mechanisms of the hypothalamopituitary axis, disrupting normal reproductive function and the menstrual cycle.

The greater degree of obesity, the more profound is the effect on the normal ovarian function.

3.7 How is fertility affected?

Fertility is reduced by the abnormal hormonal environment outlined in Q 3.6, which interferes with normal reproductive function and results in irregular and anovulatory cycles. Estimates differ, but obesity probably accounts for 6% of primary infertility, and underweight another 6% (Green et al 1988); some studies put the level of diet related infertility as high as 30%. Over 70% of women who are infertile because of body-weight anomalies will conceive spontaneously on losing weight and as little as 5% weight loss has been shown to achieve increased fertility rates. Overweight and obesity in men is also associated with infertility. The mechanism by which this occurs is less clear but infertility is probably a result of abnormal testosterone levels.

Overweight and obesity are vital factors for many infertile couples; they should be made aware that obesity can drastically reduce fertility and that regaining a healthy weight is often all that it takes to resume reproductive function. Having been informed at the earliest stage of consultation and investigation that their weight problems might be causing their infertility, patients have the chance to consider the best way forward for them, and whether losing weight – supported or on their own – is their favoured approach. Weight loss can save many couples the time, expense and distress of infertility treatment. Obesity and overweight should not be ignored in the evaluation of infertility; weight management should be considered as a first-line treatment.

Not only is a couple's fertility affected by obesity, but their chances of undergoing successful IVF treatment are also reduced. Even if IVF treatment is successful, obese women have a higher risk of complications and miscarriage. Women with a BMI 30–35 have 50% extra risk, women with BMI over 35 up to twice the risk of miscarriage (Norman et al 2001). Obese women should attempt to lose weight in a bid to become pregnant naturally or, failing that, to at least give themselves the greatest chance of succeeding with the resulting IVF procedure.

3.8 How is obesity treated in polycystic ovary syndrome?

Weight management in PCOS is similar to weight management in any condition – initially by lifestyle and dietary changes. A low-fat diet is beneficial for weight loss but a reduction in total carbohydrate as well as a switch to carbohydrates with a low glycaemic index is beneficial to help reduce the load on the pancreatic beta cells. The role of metformin in metabolic syndrome and, more specifically, PCOS is unclear. Metformin can help improve the markers of metabolic syndrome by its effect on insulin resistance. If insulin resistance is reduced then the levels of circulating insulin also decrease, causing less stimulation of the ovaries and a reduction in the production of testosterone. Some studies have been carried out the US investigating the effect of combining the drugs sibutramine and metformin to maximize the effects on weight loss.

3.9   How does obesity affect pregnancy?

Not only is it more difficult to conceive when suffering from obesity but it also makes pregnancy much more hazardous if it does occur. The risk of the mother being hospitalized during pregnancy increases four-fold in the presence of obesity. If the BMI is above 35, the risks increase to six- or seven-fold. In the US, the Surgeon General's *Call to Action on Obesity* points out that:

- Obesity during pregnancy is associated with increased risk of death in both the baby and the mother and increases the risk of maternal high blood pressure by ten times.
- In addition to many other complications, women who are obese during pregnancy are more likely to have gestational diabetes and problems with labour and delivery.
- Infants born to women who are obese during pregnancy are more likely to be high birthweight and therefore, may face a higher risk of caesarean section delivery and low blood sugar (which can be associated with brain damage and seizures).
- Obesity during pregnancy is associated with increased risk of birth defects, particularly neural tube defects such as spina bifida.

More specifically, according to a study of 100 000 primigravidae assessed between 1992 and 1996 (Baeten et al 2001), obese women were five times more likely to suffer from gestational diabetes and three times as likely to have pre-eclampsia or eclampsia. Overweight women were also nearly twice as likely to have a caesarean section than non-obese women. Unfortunately, the researchers also concluded that losing weight prior to pregnancy seems to make little difference to the outcome. Only 'not becoming obese or overweight in the first place' seems to be protective. Weight loss during the first month of pregnancy actually increases the risk of neural tube defects.

Other studies have demonstrated different complications, including increased risk of urinary tract infections and thrombophlebitis, operative risk such as increased anaesthetic, wound infection, dehiscence and thromboembolic events (Baeten et al 2001, Calandra et al 1981, Edwards et al 1978, Galtier-Dereure et al 2000, Garbaciak et al 1985, Kumari 2001).

Respiratory complications occur more in obese women during pregnancy – obstructive sleep apnoea, hypoxia and hypercapnia, which can lead to intrauterine growth retardation in the fetus, and to hypertension and increased cardiovascular risk in the mother (Vaughan et al 1976).

Other risks to the fetus include macrosomia, even in non-diabetic mothers, growth retardation, stillbirth and birth defects, including neural tube abnormalities (Hendricks et al 2001). Other congenital abnormalities include cardiac defects, orofacial clefts, club foot and abdominal wall defects. There is a three-fold increase in musculoskeletal and craniofacial abnormalities in the fetus when the pregnant mother has both obesity and diabetes. Obese mothers have twice the risk of stillbirth as well as more chance of meconium ileus, late decelerations and shoulder dystocia (Garbaciak et al 1985).

3.10 What aspects of pregnancy lead to obesity in the child?

It is well known that babies of diabetic mothers can be of exceptionally high birthweight. It is less clear whether this translates into obesity later in childhood but the offspring of obese mothers are, on average, still well above average weight after 1 year. A German study published in the *American Journal of Epidemiology* (von Kries et al 2002) revealed that maternal smoking doubled the risk of obesity in the child compared with the children of non-smoking mothers. The risk of obesity depended on the number of cigarettes smoked.

3.11 How does maternal weight-gain in pregnancy affect future likelihood of obesity in the mother?

The Institute of Medicine at the American National Academy of Sciences recommends that a normal-weight mother should expect to gain between 25 and 35 lb in pregnancy and an obese or overweight mother between 15 and 25 lb. These figures not only reflect the risk of gaining too much weight during pregnancy but also the doubts about fetal well-being if weight loss, or too little weight gain, occurs.

Women who gain too much weight during pregnancy are four times more likely to be obese a year after delivery. A study at Cornell University (Olson 2001) concluded that excessive weight gain in pregnancy is making a significant contribution to the skyrocketing levels of obesity in the US. The study looked at 577 pregnant women and found that 40% gained more than the recommended weight during gestation and that 25% of all the women were at least 10 lb heavier than the recommended weight 1 year after giving birth.

A similar study (Rooney & Schauberger 2002) looked at weight gain 6 months postpartum and found that mothers who had gained too much weight during pregnancy, and those who had failed to lose this weight after 6 months, are at a higher risk of obesity a decade later. The study also revealed that mothers who breastfeed beyond 3 months have the smallest weight gain, indicating that breastfeeding protects both mother and baby against obesity.

> This is therefore one of the fundamental issues to be tackled by governments and the medical profession if the epidemic of obesity is to be stopped.

3.12 What is the effect of obesity on the menopause?

Recent research has demonstrated that obese women, especially smokers, have more frequent and more severe episodes of hot flushes (Whiteman et al 2003). This study showed that smokers have more than double the chance of a troublesome menopause than non-smokers and that obese women with a BMI of >30 were twice as likely to be troubled by hot flushes than women with a BMI <25.

THE METABOLIC SYNDROME

3.13 What is meant by the 'deadly quartet'?

The term 'deadly quartet' is a commonly used (and inaccurate) name for the metabolic syndrome. The quartet referred to comprises obesity, insulin resistance, dyslipidaemia and hypertension but, as discussed in the following questions, there are many more than four distinctive characteristics to the syndrome. However, there is some value in the term because it emphasizes certain specific risks of the metabolic syndrome and the additional risk of coronary heart disease and stroke in obese patients.

3.14 What is the metabolic syndrome (syndrome X, insulin resistance syndrome)?

The term 'metabolic syndrome' refers to the cluster of comorbidities, often found together in obese patients, which have insulin resistance as the common denominator. The main features are impaired glucose tolerance, hypertension, dyslipidaemia, hypercoagulability and obesity. Not surprisingly, metabolic syndrome frequently leads to type 2 diabetes, cardiovascular disease and stroke, as well as many other conditions discussed below.

Metabolic syndrome was initially described in the late 1980s by Gerald Reaven, Professor of Medicine at Stanford University. Reaven (who preferred the name syndrome X, despite the mysterious connotations of the term) argued that referring to the 'metabolic syndrome' was misleading because not all the facets of the syndrome, for example hypercoagulability, are genuinely metabolic. However, the term 'insulin resistance' overlooks the fact that many of the consequences are due to the presence of *too much* insulin, rather than resistance to it. 'Metabolic syndrome' is currently the preferred term in most literature.

There is no connection between Syndrome X and cardiac syndrome X.

The WHO has defined the parameters of the metabolic syndrome as:

Hyperinsulinaemia or elevated fasting glucose or type 2 diabetes and at least two of the following: abdominal obesity, dyslipidaemia or hypertension.

Hyperinsulinaemia is defined as a fasting insulin level in the top quartile; impaired fasting glucose is defined as a fasting blood glucose between 5.6 and 6 mmol/L; diabetes is defined as a fasting blood glucose of at least 6.1 mmol/L or a previous clinical diagnosis of diabetes. Abdominal obesity is defined as a waist:hip ratio greater than 0.9 or BMI of 30+. Dyslipidaemia is defined as serum triglycerides of 1.7 mmol/L or more, high-density cholesterol (HDL) cholesterol of 1.04 mmol/L or less; and hypertension as 130/85 mmHg or greater.

The US National Heart Lung and Blood Institute (NHLBI) in America (ATP III) defines metabolic syndrome as any three of the following:

■ Abdominal obesity (defined by waist circumference): men 102 cm, women 88 cm
■ Triglycerides: ≥150 mg/dL (1.69 mmol/L)
■ HDL: men <40 mg/dL (1.0 mmol/L), women <50 mg/dL (1.3 mmol/L)
■ Blood pressure: ≥130/≥85 mmHg
■ Fasting glucose: ≥110 mg/dL (6.1 mmol/L)

3.15 What is meant by 'insulin resistance'?

Insulin is a hormone formed by the beta cells of the pancreas. It is secreted into the bloodstream and circulates to the periphery, where it stimulates the uptake of glucose by skeletal muscle. The glucose is stored in the cells and used as a source of energy. Insulin also suppresses gluconeogenesis by the liver and inhibits lipolysis (the breakdown of triglycerides, which releases fatty acids into the bloodstream) in adipose tissue.

Insulin resistance is the term used when the tissues respond sluggishly to insulin. This slow response results in increased levels of blood glucose, which requires more insulin to be produced in compensation; a condition known as hyperinsulinism.

People with metabolic syndrome have parallel insulin resistance in both the muscles and the adipose tissue, so in addition to the high insulin and glucose levels there are high levels of circulating fatty acids, leading to dyslipidaemia. In the early stages of insulin resistance these physiological changes stimulate the production of insulin, which keeps glucose levels under control but, as the situation becomes more longstanding, the feedback mechanisms become disrupted, glucose levels rise and type 2 diabetes results. In addition, the dyslipidaemia leads to cardiovascular disease. The specific lipid changes are raised triglycerides, VLDL and LDL, with a consequent reduction in HDL that results in the slow removal of chylomicrons from the blood and postprandial lipaemia.

3.16 What are the other manifestations of the metabolic syndrome and how do they occur?

In patients with insulin resistance, it is only the insulin receptors in muscle and adipose tissue that are abnormal. The other organs of the body are just as sensitive to the effects of insulin as they normally are but because of the high circulating levels of insulin in the hyperinsulinaemic state these organs become overstimulated, leading to further complications of metabolic syndrome. Reaven (see Q 3.14) described these organs as 'innocent bystanders' of the increased insulin secretion in a person with muscle and adipose insulin resistance. Among the organs affected are:

- The kidneys: which responds to insulin by retaining salt, which leads to hypertension; 50% of people with high blood pressure suffer from metabolic syndrome. The ability of the kidneys to clear uric acid is also reduced, resulting in hyperuricaemia and gout.
- The ovaries: which respond by increasing secretion of testosterone, resulting in PCOS (see Q 3.6).
- The heart: there is an increase in plasminogen activator inhibitor-1 (PAI-1, which regulates the process of fibrinolysis) resulting in hypercoagulability that further increases the risk of heart disease.
- The colon, breast, prostate gland and other organs: leading to increased cancer risk.

3.17 Does insulin resistance cause obesity?

No, but increasing degrees of obesity make the insulin resistance worse. In obese subjects there is more demand on the beta cell to produce insulin to maintain glucose homeostasis, and more adipocytes to undergo lipolysis. Not all sufferers from the metabolic syndrome are obese; it is possible to have hypertension, dyslipidaemia and impaired fasting blood sugar as a consequence of insulin resistance with a normal BMI, but obesity accentuates all the metabolic changes and is therefore pivotal to the concept of the syndrome.

3.18 What effect does insulin resistance have on the sympathetic nervous system?

The metabolic syndrome is thought to cause 'sympathetic hyperfunction', leading to higher blood pressure, a more active renin–angiotensin system, a raised pulse and, consequently, cardiovascular disease and even sudden death. The exact cause of the increased sympathetic activity is unclear but is thought to involve a number of compounds including insulin, leptin, cytokines, endorphins and non-esterified fatty acids (NEFAs), which are known to raise blood pressure, heart rate and increase α-1 adrenoceptor activity, while reducing vascular compliance (Egan 2003).

3.19 How common is the metabolic syndrome?

Not every obese person has metabolic syndrome; it is perfectly possible for an obese person to have a normal blood pressure, lipid profile, fasting blood sugar and normal insulin levels because of a normal sensitivity to insulin. However, we know from experience that many obese people have a blood pressure higher than 130/85 mmHg, with a degree of dyslipidaemia that would place them firmly in the category of metabolic syndrome. The assumption must be that a degree of insulin resistance is extremely common in the population but that only the onset of obesity causes it to be sufficiently profound to create the metabolic complications. Exactly where the line is drawn between an otherwise healthy obese individual and a sufferer from metabolic syndrome is not clear but it can be helpful to measure the fasting insulin (with the agreement of the local laboratory) because hyperinsulinism is pathognomonic of the condition. Current estimates are that 1 in 5 adults in the UK, and as many as 1 in 4 in the US, have metabolic syndrome.

Men with metabolic syndrome are more than three times more likely to die of coronary heart disease than those without it.

There are enormous ethnic differences in insulin resistance. People of non-European descent have higher insulin resistance than those of European ancestry.

3.20 What is the treatment for metabolic syndrome?

The treatment for an obese person with metabolic syndrome is weight loss, which reduces insulin resistance and brings about improvements in lipid profile, blood glucose and blood pressure (*Box 3.1*).

Treating such patients with antihypertensives, cholesterol-lowering agents, blood-thinning agents and acetylcholine esterase (ACE) inhibitors without addressing the issue of their weight is an expensive, high-risk strategy that ignores the underlying pathophysiology. Unfortunately, it is extremely common practice. It might be that weight loss in an individual is

---

BOX 3.1 The physiological benefits of a 10% weight loss

- 20–25% drop in obesity-related mortality
- 30–40% drop in diabetes-related mortality
- 40–50% drop in obesity-related cancer deaths
- 10 mmHg drop in both systolic and diastolic blood pressure
- > 50% reduction in the risk of developing diabetes
- 30–50% drop in fasting glucose
- 15% drop in HbA1c
- 10% drop in total cholesterol
- 15% drop in LDL
- 30% drop in triglycerides
- 8% increase in HDL

---

impossible or insufficient, or that even marked weight loss alone does not completely restore metabolic factors to normal. In these instances, treatment for one or more individual component of the metabolic syndrome, e.g. blood pressure, might be necessary. In other instances, pharmacotherapy might be required as an intermediate measure while weight loss is being accomplished. As a rule, the management of each individual component of the metabolic syndrome is no different to the management of that condition in isolation; that is, the treatment of raised cholesterol is the same, with or without the presence of metabolic syndrome. The exception is that in the treatment of blood pressure, diuretics should be used with caution because of the effects of high circulating insulin on the kidneys, and β-blockers should be avoided if possible because of the chance of weight gain.

The study of metabolic syndrome acts as a clear illustration to clinicians who do not consider treating obesity as essential, or do not believe it is an important chronic medical condition. Regardless of the underlying cause, obesity must be treated as a priority because of the sinister metabolic sequelae.

3.21 How should weight loss be brought about in metabolic syndrome?

Weight loss should be attempted in the usual way, starting with diet, exercise and lifestyle changes, with second-line treatments such as pharmacotherapy being used as necessary. However, the dietary guidelines are slightly complicated by the presence of insulin resistance. The diet should be low in fat to induce weight loss but should contain a certain amount of unsaturates and monosaturates, for example from oily fish, to improve the lipid profile. As excess carbohydrate has the potential to increase insulin secretion and overload the system, putting more pressure on the beta cells and worsening all the metabolic effects of the syndrome, the recommendation is to:

- ■ Reduce the fat content of the diet, in particular avoiding saturated fats.
- ■ Maintain or reduce the carbohydrate content of the diet, favouring high-fibre, low-glycaemic-index foods that have a relatively benign effect on the insulin system.
- ■ Reduce dietary intake of salt to avoid aggravating the effect of insulin on the renal system.

HYPERTENSION

3.22 What is the extent of the link between obesity and hypertension?

There is a very close link between obesity, particularly abdominal obesity, and hypertension; it has been reported that up to two-thirds of cases of hypertension are linked with obesity (Cassano et al 1990). Obese people have over five times the normal risk of developing hypertension (Wolf & Colditz 1998) and people who are 20% overweight are eight times more likely to develop the condition (Pi-Sunyer 1993). In fact, obesity has been described as the major modifiable correlate of blood pressure (Havlik et al 1983).

The Framingham study (McMahon et al 1987) demonstrated that every 4.5-kg increase in weight led to a gain of around 4.3 mmHg systolic blood pressure, and that a 15% gain in weight was associated with an 18% increase in systolic blood pressure.

3.23 What is the relationship between obesity and hypertension?

The exact cause of the association is unclear and there are known to be multiple factors. One such factor is the raised insulin level (which occurs with the metabolic syndrome), which has a stimulant effect on the kidneys, leading to salt retention and hypertension.

Another factor could be sleep apnoea, which causes hypertension as a result of prolonged hypoxia and by changes in thoracic pressure. The collapse of the pharyngeal airway that occurs in sleep apnoea results in increased respiratory effort and increasingly negative intrathoracic pressure, until hypoxia causes arousal from sleep and normal service is resumed.

Many other phenomena associated with obesity also predispose to hypertension or potentiate the effects of hypertension, leading to coronary heart disease. These include left ventricular hypertrophy, increased coagulability, interference with the sympathetic nervous system and dyslipidaemia.

Blood pressure must be measured with a cuff that is large enough to embrace 80% of the upper arm, otherwise an abnormally high reading will result. Such a cuff should be readily available so that neither patient nor doctor is embarrassed by a search.

3.24 How does weight loss improve hypertension?

It has been shown that weight loss not only induces a reduction in blood pressure but that it also prevents hypertension in at-risk normotensive people (Blackburn 1995). Weight loss of 10% has been demonstrated to cause reduction of blood pressure of between 10 and 20 mmHg systolic and diastolic (see Box 3.1). Jung (1997) demonstrated a reduction of 1 mmHg systolic and 2 mmHg diastolic for each 1% reduction in weight (see http://www.ccjm.org/pdffiles/Nambi1202.pdf and http://www.metabolicsyndromeonline.com/Monograph.pdf).

3.25 How is hypertension in obesity treated?

Blood pressure will often need treatment with antihypertensive medication at the same time as weight loss is occurring, although treatment can be temporary if sufficient weight loss is induced. Beta-blockers should be avoided because of the risk of weight gain and it is suggested that thiazide and other diuretics should be avoided because of the renal-induced salt imbalance.

DYSLIPIDAEMIA

3.26 What is the risk of dyslipidaemia?

There is a strong association between obesity and raised cholesterol. LDL cholesterol becomes raised, the protective HDL cholesterol is reduced and triglyceride levels, which are a high-risk marker for cerebrovascular disease, are increased (Fig. 3.1). The mechanism for these changes derives from the insulin resistance of adipose tissue, resulting in decreased levels of lipoprotein lipase and hence raised LDL and disordered fat metabolism. It is estimated that around 38% of patients with a BMI >27 suffer from hypercholesterolaemia (Hoffman-La Roche, data on file). The Framingham study revealed that cholesterol increased by 12 mg/dL for every 10% weight gain. Conversely, weight loss can be shown to improve lipid profile. The American National Cholesterol Education Programme reported that for every 3 kg of diet-induced weight lost, HDL increases by 1 mg/dL; and it is widely accepted that a 10% weight loss will induce a reduction in LDL of approximately 15%, and increase in HDL of 8%, with a 10% fall in total cholesterol (RCP).

Pharmacotherapy for obesity has been shown to improve dyslipidaemias in obese patients on drugs plus lifestyle management. Orlistat has been

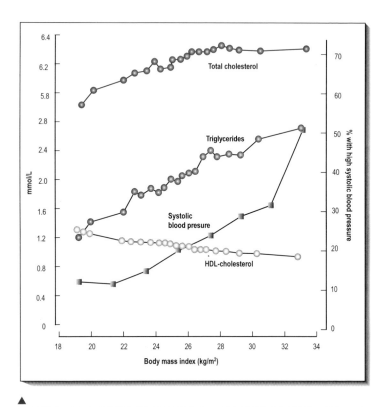

▲

Fig. 3.1 Body mass index (BMI) is related to higher levels of total cholesterol, triglycerides and systolic blood pressure, and to a decreased level of HDL-cholesterol, all of which are risk factors for disease (data derived from Shaper et al 1991).

shown to reduce total and LDL cholesterol and increase the HDL:LDL ratio (Rossner et al 2000) and Fujioka et al (2000) demonstrated the beneficial effects of sibutramine on lipid profiles. Trials with phentermine and dexfenfluramine have also shown benefits on lipid profile (Bremer et al 1994, Weintraub et al 1992).

CARDIOVASCULAR DISEASE

3.27 How does obesity affect cardiovascular risk?

Coronary heart disease (CHD) is one of the most common causes of excess illness and death in obese people because of the potent combined effects of raised blood pressure, high cholesterol, physical inactivity and type 2 diabetes. Hypertension, myocardial infarction, stroke and congestive cardiac failure are all significantly more common in obesity; left ventricular size and wall thickness increase with BMI (Lavie et al 1992) because of increased cardiac output. As with other risk factors, abdominal or 'android' obesity is associated with higher risk than 'gynoid' obesity. The increased levels of LDL cholesterol and triglycerides lead to the enhanced formation of atheromatous plaques in the blood vessels; this factor, combined with the increased coagulability of the blood (*see Q 3.14*) leads to the increased risk of arterial occlusion (Meade et al 1993). There is a three-fold increase in risk of a fatal or non-fatal MI in women with BMI >29 compared with their leaner counterparts. The Nurses Health study (Colditz et al 1990) demonstrated similar figures in women: double the risk of CHD in BMI 25–29 and 3.6 times the risk in women with BMI >29. The Framingham study (Herbert et al 1983) confirms the link between obesity and CHD, and suggests that increasing weight during adulthood might have the greatest impact on CHD; in technical terms, it demonstrated that the risk of heart disease increases by 15% in men and 22% in women for every standard deviation increase in weight.

Although weight loss reduces the risk of heart disease and stroke, the fact that plaque has already been formed and laid down within the arteries suggests that there is likely to still be an increased cardiovascular risk even after weight loss has occurred. The finding of high cholesterol levels and hypertension in obese children as young as 9 has led to the concept of childhood obesity 'casting a shadow' on future health, and increasing morbidity and mortality in adulthood, even if the obesity itself is remedied.

3.28 How does this affect clinical practice?

In practice, it is important to make an accurate assessment of cardiovascular risk by using, for instance, Framingham or Sheffield tables. However, obesity was not considered important enough by the Framingham investigators to be given the status of 'independent risk factor', although it was measured accurately during the study. This could be because of the relatively low prevalence of the condition when the study was conducted (in the mid- to late 1980s) compared with today's epidemic. Whatever the reason, it does diminish the usefulness of the tables when considering the cardiovascular risk of an obese person. It is reassuring for doctor and patient alike to see the cardiac risk factors tumble as weight is reduced, and other parameters, for example, blood pressure and cholesterol, follow suit.

3.29 Is there a link between obesity and cardiac arrhythmias?

There are various reasons why obesity can cause arrhythmias, including hypoxia, hypercapnia, coronary artery disease, sleep apnoea, myocardial hypertrophy and fatty infiltration of the conducting system (Adams & Murphy 2000).

3.30 What is the association between obesity and stroke?

The incidence of stroke is increased in the presence of obesity, although the relationship is less clear than in the case of heart disease. It seems self-evident that the risk of stroke in obesity is increased because of the simultaneous presence of dyslipidaemia and hypertension, but it is an area that has not been closely studied. The Northern Manhattan Stroke Study (Suk et al 2003) concluded that abdominal obesity is an independent, potent risk factor for ischaemic stroke in all ethnic groups. A waist:hip ratio in the highest quartile was associated with a risk ratio of 3 (adjusted for other risk factors) in men and women of all ethnic groups, but the effect was most pronounced in young people.

3.31 How much heart disease is caused by obesity?

Increased insulin resistance caused by obesity often leads to a dyslipidaemic state, macrovascular atheroma formation, endothelial dysfunction and microvascular complications. Similarly, with the increased risk of hypertensive disease, cardiovascular disease is much more common in obese individuals.

According to National Audit Office estimates:

- the increased risk of an obese adult developing hypertension is 4.2-fold in women and 2.6-fold in men
- the increased risk of myocardial infarction of 3.2 in women and 1.5 in men
- the increased risk of angina of 1.8 in both men and women.

In terms of causality, it has been stated that obesity is responsible for 17% of all cardiovascular disease. In other words, if obesity were wholly prevented or treated, 17% of cardiovascular cases would be prevented. In Canada in 1997 it was estimated that cardiovascular disease accounted for 54% of the direct costs of obesity. In primary care, almost one-third of cardiovascular patients have been found to be clinically obese.

ASTHMA

3.32 What is the link between asthma and obesity?

It is well known that there is a connection between obesity and asthma but the more research is published on the subject, the more difficult it seems to be to pin-down the exact association. Certain alterations in respiratory function are unsurprising and well documented in obesity, for instance a reduced total lung capacity, reduced residual volume and functional residual capacity but it is more difficult to evaluate other contributory changes, or to prove the underlying cause of breathlessness.

3.33 What is the conflicting evidence?

One study published in the *Journal of Asthma* (Brenner et al 2001) compared a group of asthmatic children with a group of children without asthma and found that 17% of the non-asthmatic children were obese, compared with 20% of the asthmatic children; an insignificant difference, suggesting no link between overweight and asthma. However, a much larger, 5-year study at Harvard University (Camargo et al 1999) looked at 85 911 nurses (of whom 1652 suffered from asthma) discovered that those with obesity were 2.7 times more likely to have asthma.

Two reports published in *Thorax* (Chinn & Rona 2001, von Mutuis et al 2001) came to conflicting conclusions. One revealed that increasing rates of asthma are linked to the obesity epidemic, and that the heaviest children were 77% more likely to have wheezing and shortness of breath, whereas the other pointed out that asthma incidence has been increasing for decades and that the obesity epidemic is too recent a phenomenon to explain this satisfactorily.

The British Thoracic Society suggests that 'the jury is still out on the link between obesity and asthma in childhood', pointing out that asthma can occur in people of all sizes. More research is needed to discover whether – if there genuinely *is* a relationship between the two – the lack of physical exercise due to poorly controlled airways disease leads to obesity or if it is the physical effects of airway obstruction and upwards pressure from the belly on the diaphragm in obese patients, which contributes to the asthma.

3.34 What are the possible reasons why asthma and obesity coexist?

The incidences of both obesity and asthma are increasing at an alarming rate. This could simply be that both conditions have the same root causes in twenty-first century life. It has been suggested that the common denominator is 'urban sprawl': the increase in built-up areas around towns, leading to more car use, more sedentary behaviour, less physical activity and more pollution; all of which predisposes the same people to both conditions. Also breast-feeding, which protects children against both conditions, is still at an unacceptably low level in the UK, which could result in a high coexisting incidence of both conditions. Recent theories allege that children who have reduced contact with dirt and common allergens at an early age have a greater risk of asthma; as obesity is present in the same population in epidemic proportions there is bound to be a degree of overlap.

Researchers in Cincinatti (American Academy of Allergy, Asthma and Immunology 2003) reported the discovery of a gene, RELM-b, which is linked to insulin resistance and asthma in mice, and have suggested this as a possible causal link in humans.

Other reports (Sin et al 2002) argue that although obesity is certainly linked with shortness of breath, this isn't necessarily due to asthma or to airflow obstruction. In their study of 16 000 participants, those with increasing levels of obesity reported more physical restrictions and limitations than their leaner counterparts in, for instance, walking up a hill, but the participants with higher BMI were actually less likely to suffer from significant airflow obstruction. The researchers concluded that the cause of dyspnoea was more likely to be respiratory mechanics and gas exchange. Put simply, obese people become short of breath because they have more to carry around. The importance of this finding is that obese, dyspnoeic but non-asthmatic patients might be wrongly diagnosed and treated with inappropriate, expensive and potentially dangerous drugs.

DIABETES

3.35 How much diabetes is caused by obesity?

Impaired glucose tolerance and type 2 diabetes are often caused directly by the physiological effects of overweight and obesity. Of course, there are many obese non-diabetic individuals, but in those who are genetically susceptible to type 2 diabetes, development of obesity markedly increases the risk of frank diabetes. This should come as no surprise given that 85% of type 2 diabetics are overweight or obese.

3.36 How strong is the connection between obesity and type 2 diabetes?

The connection between obesity and type 2 diabetes is so strong, that attempting to treat diabetes properly without managing any coexisting obesity is almost futile. The association between the conditions is so close that many experts consider obesity and type 2 diabetes to be different ends of the same spectrum, and that obesity should be treated as a prediabetic condition. The term 'diabesity' is increasingly being used.

The reason for the link is explored under metabolic syndrome (*see* Q 3.14), in particular the fact that insulin resistance, which is the primary defect in type 2 diabetes, is also the fundamental problem in the metabolic syndrome.

A famous study by Sims et al (1973) took normal young men with no family history of type 2 diabetes and overfed them for 6 months, increasing their average body weight by 21% to a BMI of 28. This resulted in increased fasting insulin, glucose, triglycerides and an impaired glucose tolerance, which returned to baseline levels when feeding returned to normal.

Statistics emphasize the point; 85–90% of 'diabetics' have type 2 diabetes and approximately 80–85% of type 2 diabetics are obese; a staggering 12% of people with a BMI >27 have type 2 diabetes. In men, a waist circumference of over 100 cm increases the risk of diabetes 3.5-fold (Chan et al 1994). The relative risks compared to a person with a BMI of 22 are shown in *Fig. 3.2*.

In other words, during a normal Monday morning surgery, a patient with BMI of 35 is 93 times more likely to develop type 2 diabetes than the lean person who has the next appointment. There are estimated to be over one million undiagnosed diabetics in the UK, giving a high probability that this particular obese patient is either one of the missing million or soon will be, and an absolute certainty that sooner rather than later some of the obese patients on a particular doctor's books will become diabetic.

The National Health and Nutrition Examination Study (NHANES; Ford et al 1997) demonstrates that for each kilogram of weight gain in the population the risk of diabetes rises by an impressive 4.5%.

3.37 What are the risks of type 2 diabetes?

The risks of type 2 diabetes are well documented; coronary heart disease, dyslipidaemia, blindness, renal failure, amputation and so on. Failing to diagnose the condition, and thus missing the opportunity to prevent the sequelae, is a costly error and an illustration that obesity must not be

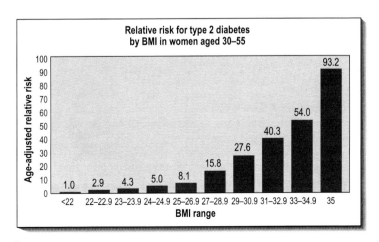

Fig. 3.2 Relative risk for type 2 diabetes by BMI in women aged 30–55 (data derived from Colditz et al 1995).

ignored; 10% of NHS resources are spent on diabetes and its complications, on behalf of only 3% of the population. WHO fact sheet 138 (revised April 2002) describes diabetes as the most important consequence of obesity. There are currently estimated to be over 150 million cases worldwide, a number that is likely to double by 2025 (*see Q 1.12*).

One of the most disturbing aspects of the increasing numbers of people with type 2 diabetes is the fact that adult-onset diabetes is now being seen in children as young as 10. Until recently, type 2 diabetes was unknown in children – it was usually restricted to adults over the age of 40. However, because of the increasing levels of childhood obesity it is now being seen in grossly obese children (weighing 20 stone or more). Although the phenomenon was initially reported in the US, the first cases of childhood-onset type 2 diabetes are being seen in the UK. Children such as these have a whole lifetime in which to develop the complications of diabetes, not to mention the comorbidities of obesity itself. Their shortened life expectancy has made some commentators believe that the current generation will be the first in which parents consistently outlive their children.

3.38 How does losing weight help to treat diabetes?

Weight loss is a vital part of diabetes treatment. A 10% loss of weight will result in an improvement of all the markers for diabetes, and in many cases will enable patients to avoid resorting to, for instance, antihypertensives and hypoglycaemic agents. *Box 3.1* (p. 43) highlights the benefits of a 10% weight loss.

A study in 1995 (Williamson et al 1995) showed that weight loss of 0.5–9.0 kg is associated with a 30–40% reduction in diabetes-related mortality.

Many diabetics will need pharmacotherapy to control their diabetes in addition to losing weight, but it is clear that weight loss is an integral part of diabetes management, without which diabetes treatment cannot be 100% successful. It is therefore essential that all diabetic patients are weighed, have their height measured and have their waist circumference recorded. They must be given dietary and lifestyle advice for weight management as well as for glycaemic control.

3.39 What is the best pharmacotherapy for diabetes?

The hypoglycaemic drug of choice in obese or overweight diabetics is metformin, because of its beneficial effect on insulin resistance. It can help patients lose weight, and bring about a reduction in all the risk factors associated with insulin resistance and metabolic syndrome.

Other hypoglycaemics, such as the sulphonylureas and glitazones, and even insulin, have weight gain as a side-effect. If such drugs are necessary for glycaemic control, patients should be warned of the deleterious effect on their weight, and weight management efforts redoubled.

Pharmacotherapy for obesity will often be appropriate for obese type 2 diabetics and has been shown to be successful in improving the markers of the condition. One study (Fujioki et al 2000) looked at obese patients with poorly controlled type 2 diabetes and concluded that:

Sibutramine produced statistically and clinically significant weight loss when used in combination with recommendations for moderate caloric restriction. This weight loss was associated with improvements in metabolic control and quality of life, and sibutramine was generally well tolerated in obese patients with type 2 diabetes.

In the Fujioki et al (2000) study, 33% of patients achieved weight loss of $\geq$5%, and 8% of patients achieved a weight loss of 10%. HbA_1c was reduced by 0.53 and 1.65, respectively, in the 5 and 10% responders and fasting glucose dropped by 1.4 mmol/L and 3.8 mmol/L, respectively.

Orlistat was the subject of the XENDOS trial (*see Q 7.28*), which demonstrated that the risk of developing type 2 diabetes in obese subjects was 37% lower in people treated with orlistat when compared to lifestyle intervention alone, and patients treated with orlistat benefited from long-term improvements in cardiovascular risk factors such as blood pressure and lipid profiles.

CANCER

3.40 What is the link between obesity and cancer?

Obesity is the biggest preventable cause of cancer after smoking. Considering this fact, there is a dearth of scientific research, information in the medical journals, publicity in the lay press or action in parliament to reflect the problem. Compared with the coverage given to smoking-related cancer and breast cancer, and the financial resources that go with this, obesity is a very poor second, despite its massive importance.

Obesity carries a high financial and human cost but, unlike smoking-related cancer and breast cancer, we are currently seeing only the tip of the iceberg of obesity-related cancer. The future figures will inevitably mirror the predicted rise in adult obesity.

The exact cause of the association is not known in all cases but the statistics on prevalence, as well as the mortality and morbidity rates, suggest that research, awareness and intervention must be carried out enthusiastically if the rising tide of obesity isn't to be accompanied by a cancer epidemic.

It has been well documented for years that certain cancers have a raised incidence in obese people, and cancers such as endometrial cancer are almost exclusively restricted to the obese. The causal relationship is not always completely understood and differs from one form of cancer to another. Recent advances and population studies, however, have started to shed more light on the physiological and biochemical basis of the disease.

3.41 What is the risk of obese people getting cancer?

In February 2002, the International Agency for Research on Cancer estimated that overweight and inactivity accounts for one-quarter to one-third of cases of breast cancer, colon cancer, endometrial cancer, kidney cancer and oesophageal cancer. *Box 3.2* shows those cancers that are associated with obesity. The increased risk varies between the different sorts of cancer. For instance, cancer of the colon has a risk ratio of 2.7 in women and 3.0 in men, and ovarian cancer is 1.7 times more likely in obese women.

Obesity in patients more than 40% overweight carries an overall mortality ratio for cancer of 1.55 in men and 1.33 in women (Garfinkel 1985); the same women are 5.4 times as likely to get endometrial cancer.

It is estimated that 10% of all cancer deaths among non-smokers are obesity related.

A Swedish study (Wolk et al 2001) followed 28 000 obese patients for up to 29 years. The increased incidence of cancer was 33% compared to the general population, with a breakdown of 25% among men and 37% among women. As well as the previously well-documented associations with cancer, this study also suggested a link with cancer of the larynx, small bowel and non-Hodgkin's lymphoma.

A study published in the *New England Journal of Medicine* (Chow et al 2000) of the records of over 360 000 Swedish men revealed that obese men had almost double the risk of renal cell cancer.

BOX 3.2 Cancers risk and obesity
Obesity increases the risk of the following cancers:

- breast
- colon
- prostate
- testicle
- endometrium
- liver
- cervix
- ovary
- kidney
- gall bladder
- oesophagus
- pancreas
- Hodgkin's disease

3.42 What causes cancer in obese patients?

The exact cause of the different forms of cancer are not fully understood but the rise in obesity-related cancers is directly associated with those changes found in the metabolic syndrome. In fact, it would not be unreasonable to suggest that increased cancer risk should be added to the list of morbidities that comprise the metabolic syndrome.

The fundamental defect in metabolic syndrome is insulin resistance – the sluggish reaction of cells in muscle and adipose tissue to the actions of insulin. This results in increased levels of blood glucose and, to compensate, increased levels of circulating insulin; this condition is known as hyperinsulinaemia (*see* Q 3.14).

However, other organs are not resistant to the action of insulin and display a heightened response to the high levels of insulin (and possibly other insulin-like hormones that act as growth factors). The result of this overstimulation is more rapid cell turnover, therefore a greater cancer risk. Adipose tissue also secretes oestrogen (*see* Q 3.44), which, combined with insulin, forms a potent carcinogenic mixture.

3.43 What is the link between cancer of the colon and obesity?

Cancer of the colon, the third most common cancer in the US, is a multifactorial condition caused partly by genetic factors and partly by environmental factors, for instance smoking. Obesity is thought to have two effects, which combine to make colonic cancer more common. One is that adipose tissue traps dietary and environmental carcinogens, which would otherwise be excreted; the other is increased cell turnover as a result of excess levels of insulin.

3.44 What is the link between renal cancer and obesity?

Renal cancer is more common in obesity – more so in women than men. This is possibly a result of the combination of oestrogen with excess insulin. The action of insulin on the kidney also increases salt retention, leading to hypertension.

3.45 What is the link between breast cancer and obesity?

Breast cancer is one of the hormone-sensitive malignancies and has been widely linked with oestrogens – both natural and in the combined contraceptive pill and hormone replacement therapy. In obese women, not only is there an abnormally high level of oestrogen, caused by peripheral conversion of androgens in adipose tissue, but this high level is maintained in the postmenopausal state because fat cells continue to secrete oestrogens long after the ovaries have ceased. Therefore, in obese women it is thought that prolonged exposure to carcinogenic hormones after the menopause is a contributory factor to the higher prevalence of breast cancer. It is also thought that the growth factor effect of insulin combines with the hormonal influence to potentiate the effect.

3.46 What is the link between endometrial cancer and obesity?

Endometrial cancer is the fourth most common cancer in women. The endometrium is acted upon by higher levels of oestrogen, for longer, in the same way as the breast. It is well recognized that non-hysterectomized patients should not receive unopposed oestrogens for risk of causing endometrial hyperplasia and malignancy; oestrogen secreted by the adipose tissues mimics such unopposed oestrogen, hence the danger.

3.47 What is the link between prostate cancer and obesity?

Cancer of the prostate is the most common male cancer. It has an increased prevalence in obesity as a result of the combined actions of insulin and an abnormal hormone profile. Just as giving testosterone to a patient with hypogonadism disturbs the natural hormonal balance, increasing the risk of prostate cancer, so the abnormal levels of the hormone in obesity have a similar effect.

3.48 What is the link between oesophageal cancer and obesity?

Cancer of the oesophagus in obesity has a completely different aetiology than in non-obese individuals. It is thought to be caused by an increase in gastric reflux of acid, which in the result of increased pressure on the stomach contents from an obese abdomen (for details, see All American Institute of Cancer Research: www.aicr.org).

3.49 How can obesity-related cancer be combated?

Weight management is the key to prevention of obesity-related cancers, but there are also specific recommendations relevant to certain conditions.

Because of the effect of prolonged high levels of oestrogen on the breast and endometrium in obese women it is important to avoid gaining weight during adult life, in particular middle age. This also seems to reduce the possibility of a build-up of carcinogens in fatty tissue, which is part of the pathogenesis of colonic cancer. A diet high in vegetables, fruit wholegrains and beans is probably protective. The American Institute of Cancer Research cites physical exercise as being of particular importance in reducing the risks of obesity-related cancer, although the paucity of research makes it difficult to pin down the exact mechanism. It is suggested that lifelong regular exercise decreases the effect of prolonged insulin exposure.

At a meeting in February 2001, the International Agency for Research on Cancer (part of the WHO) concluded that overweight and a sedentary lifestyle are associated with raised cancer risk and recommended that, to minimize the risk, overweight and obese people should avoid gaining extra weight and should lose weight through dietary changes and exercise.

ARTHRITIS

3.50 What is the link between obesity and osteoarthritis?

There is a well-documented link between obesity and osteoarthritis, although the cause is not completely clear. It is often assumed that the connection between lower-limb arthritis and excess body weight is merely due to the increased load these susceptible joints have to support, usually over many years. But it has also been suggested that damage to the joint surface is due to a metabolic effect, caused by the release of cytokines from adipose tissue (see Q 2.18) having a direct inflammatory action leading to arthritis. A cohort of the Framingham study (Felson et al 1988) looked at the relative risk of radiographic osteoarthritis of the knee for various weight groups, adjusted for age, physical activity and uric acid levels. It was discovered that women in the heaviest quintile for weight had more than double the risk of osteoarthritis in the knee, whereas men had 1.5 times the risk, but the precise cause of the condition was not postulated. A study at St Thomas' Hospital (Cicuttini et al 1996) found a link between obesity and osteoarthritis of the carpometacarpal joints of the hand, which suggests a metabolic cause because these joints are non-weight-bearing. Van Saase et al (1988) found that obesity was clearly associated with osteoarthritis in all those joints most frequently affected, whether or not they were weight bearing. This implies a metabolic cause and, although not offering an explanation, does suggest the scope for prevention of osteoarthritis by weight loss.

A recent paper (Jordan et al 2002) demonstrated a link between symptomatic spinal osteoarthritis and low birthweight, but also concluded that the problem is worse in those who were low birthweight babies but went on to become overweight as adults. This suggests that weight *gain* is an important aetiological factor in the condition. A second study on the effects of changing weight revealed that increased weight in women, but not men, was linked to worsening of symptoms of knee osteoarthritis, whereas a reduction of 10% weight by men, but not women, resulted in a significant reduction in symptoms (Lethbridge-Cejku et al 2002).

The most common explanation is backed by the NHANES study, which concluded that there is a link between osteoarthritis and obesity, and that additional mechanical stress is the cause.

3.51 Should obese patients be offered joint replacements if they don't lose weight?

Research shows that obese patients enjoy as much improvement from joint replacement as anyone else after knee and hip replacements (Stickles et al 2001). Enabling obese patients who have previously been unable to exercise to increase their level of physical activity, and therefore prevent the comorbidities of obesity, is a persuasive argument in favour of joint replacement surgery in the obese. In practice, however, it is reported to be 'unusual for obese patients to lose weight following arthroplasty, despite promises to the contrary' (Vazquez-Vela Johnson et al 2003).The same authors demonstrated that obese patients produced excessive demands on their total knee replacements, especially men under 60, leading to a 10-year 'survival' rate in this group of only 35.7%.

GOUT

3.52 What is the link between obesity and gout?

There is known to be a link between obesity and gout, hyperuricaemia being one of the changes ascribed to the metabolic syndrome. Japanese Sumo wrestlers seem to be particularly prone to gout and have been found to have high levels of uric acid, which increase as BMI increases (WHO 2000). A study in Massachusetts in 2002 (Choi et al 2002) revealed a strong link between weight gain in men after the age of 21 and the chance of developing gout, which supported the findings of previous reports. However, more research is needed to ascertain whether, for instance, high alcohol intake or other factors cause both conditions. The eighteenth-century physician and celebrated wit George Cheyne wrote of 'inveterate *Gouts* and decay'd *Constitutions*' in whom 'the *Intemperance* and Groffnefs in diet, and the *Inactivity* of the *People*' lead to the condition (although in the early 1700s the term 'gout' could be applied to all manner of ailments).

ACCIDENTAL INJURY

3.53 What is the association between obesity and accidental injury?

There is an increased risk of accidental injury in obese subjects. This may be predominantly a result of decreased mobility, balance problems, increased inertia on movement and the fact that obese people are likely to be less nimble in avoiding dangerous situations. William Banting, the obese author of *Letter on Corpulence Addressed to the Public* in 1864 – the first commercially available diet – was 'compelled to go downstairs slowly backwards, to save the jar of increased weight upon the ancle [sic] and knee joints, and been obliged to puff and blow with every slight exertion'. Another major factor, however, is sleep apnoea, which results in daytime somnolence and increased risk of road traffic accidents. Sufferers from sleep apnoea have two to three times the risk of car accidents and 5–7 times the risk of multiple accidents (see http://www.healthandage.com/Home/gm=6!gid6=6505).

A study reported in the journal *Sleep* (Stoohs et al 1994) looked at long-distance haulage drivers and found a strong link between sleep apnoea sufferers and driving accidents, but also discovered that obese drivers with a body mass ≥ 30 kg/m^2 also presented a two-fold higher accident rate than non-obese drivers. Obese victims of traffic accidents are more likely to suffer fractures, especially of ribs, pelvis and extremities, but are less likely to suffer liver damage or head injury (Adams & Murphy 2000).

SKIN DISORDERS

3.54 What is the link between obesity and skin disorders?

Diabetes is well known to cause many different dermatological conditions, including necrobiosis lipoidica, acanthosis nigricans, ulcers and infections. Obesity coexisting with diabetes will aggravate these conditions, many of which can occur in the non-diabetic obese patient. Dr George Cheyne, the eighteenth-century physician, celebrity and behemoth overindulged to the extent that 'every dinner necessarily became a Surfeit and a Debauch' until his legs 'broke out all over in scorbutick ulcers' and he suffered various attacks of erysipelas. Chronic varicose ulcers are commonplace in the obese, especially the elderly, along with dependent oedema and 'poor circulation'. Common infections such as thrush and intertrigo and erysipelas are more prevalent in obesity, and even necrotizing fasciitis has a higher prevalence in obese subjects. Certain skin lesions such as xanthelasmata and papillomata are more common with obesity.

3.55 What is the effect of obesity on the blood?

Obesity causes increased fibrinogen, decreased plasminogen activator, elevated plasminogen activator inhibitor-1 (PAI-1) and increased blood viscosity as part of the metabolic syndrome. The formation of atherosclerotic plaques is increased, as is the size of the thrombus following plaque rupture. Other dangerous haematological changes that occur in obesity include enhanced activation of endothelial cells, promotion of LDL oxidation, increased platelet aggregation, activation of factor VII and an increase in prothrombin and in factors IX and X.

As well as adding to the risk of stroke and coronary heart disease, this hypercoagulability leads to increased prevalence of deep vein thrombosis, especially if mobility is impaired. George Cheyne's blood was 'one impenetrable *Mass* of *Glew*' with 'every *Vein* and *Artery* like so many Black Puddings'.

GALL BLADDER DISEASE

3.56 What is the connection between obesity and gallstones?

The fact that gallstones are more prevalent in people who are 'female, fair, forty and fat ' is well known. Gall bladder disease is undoubtedly more common in females and the evidence is increasing that obesity is a major contributing factor. The risk of gallstones increases three-fold in women with BMI >32 compared with those with a BMI of 25, and seven-fold in women with BMI >45. The risk increases to 20 per 1000 women per year with BMI ≥40 (see http://www.nhlbi.nih.gov/guidelines/obesity/e_txtbk/). The increased prevalence is associated with the higher levels of serum cholesterol, often in association with a large dysfunctional gall bladder and, in instances of low-fat diets, a reduced frequency of gall bladder contractions.

There is particular risk of gallstone formation in patients who lose weight rapidly, by dieting or other means, including surgical. Gallstone formation after surgery has been observed at levels of up to 38% (Shiffman et al 1992; see also http://www.obesity-online.com/gallengl.htm) and some centres even carry out prophylactic cholecystectomy along with bariatric procedures, despite the technical difficulty of such operations in obese patients. Use of prophylactic drugs such as ursodeoxycholic acid to prevent stone formation is also increasingly common.

Rapid weight loss by dieting has been shown to cause gallstones, as well as causing silent gallstones to become symptomatic; a weight loss of above 3 lb/week is thought to increase the risk. Between 10 and 25% of patients on VLCD might develop gallstones (http://www.weight-loss-i.com/gallstones-weight-obesity.htm), approximately one-third of whom develop symptoms. 'Yo-yo' dieting is thought to substantially increase the risk of gall bladder disease, especially with fluctuations of 10 lb or more in either direction.

Prevention of gallstones is assisted by gradual weight loss, with a moderate but significant amount of fat in the diet, with high fibre and calcium, in the presence of increased physical exercise.

Gall bladder cancer is also more prevalent in obese people than in the non-obese.

LIVER DISEASE

3.57 What is the association between obesity and liver disease?

As well as causing gall bladder disease, obesity is linked with fatty changes within the liver. It has been recognized for some time that changes in liver function tests associated with fatty accumulation within the liver occur with obesity, usually have a benign prognosis and fall within the description of non-alcoholic fatty liver disease (NAFLD).

Recently, however, non-alcoholic steatohepatitis (NASH) – a much more serious sequel to benign fatty liver – is increasingly being recognized. NASH is becoming more and more prevalent in Western society and is important because of its likely progression to cirrhosis, portal hypertension and even hepatocellular carcinoma. It is set to become one of the most prevalent causes of end-stage liver disease in the developed world (Khedr & Elias 2003) and it has been said to be the most common cause of persistently abnormal liver function tests after hepatitis C (Day 2002).

The dramatic changes in liver histology classically seen in alcoholic hepatitis are typical of NASH, but instead of alcohol being involved the aetiological factors are obesity, diabetes, hyperlipidaemia and hypertension, placing it firmly within the definition of the metabolic syndrome (*see* Q 3.14). Obesity is thought to be the main cause and insulin resistance is a key factor in its aetiology; patients with NASH have been shown to be more insulin resistant than those with benign fatty liver alone (Day 2002). As with metabolic syndrome, it is possible to suffer from NASH without being obese; the condition is also increasingly prevalent in children.

3.58   How is NASH diagnosed?

NASH usually occurs in obese middle-aged people who often have diabetes, an abnormal lipid profile or hypertension. Symptoms might be non-existent, although some patients may complain of tiredness and abdominal discomfort; hepatomegaly occurs in up to 75% of patients, but other signs of liver disease are rare (de Knegt 2001). The finding of raised levels of gamma glutamyl transferase (γ-GT), alanine transaminase (ALT) and, to a lesser extent, aspartate transaminase (AST) and alkaline phosphatase, might be the first indications of NAFLD and could be associated with an abnormally echogenic 'white' or 'bright' appearance of the liver on ultrasound. Although CT and MRI can demonstrate gross hepatic steatosis, liver biopsy is the 'gold standard' diagnostic test, revealing identical features to alcoholic liver disease. However, the invasive nature of liver biopsy limits its use in practice. The extent to which NAFLD and NASH are different stages of the same illness is still unclear, as is how progression from one to the other occurs. The prevalence of NASH in the general population is estimated to be between 2% and 9%, of whom 50% will develop fibrosis, 30% will develop cirrhosis and 3% end up with liver failure or transplantation.

3.59   What is the cause of NASH?

NASH is now generally viewed as part of the metabolic syndrome and is specifically associated with visceral obesity. Visceral adipocytes are known to be more insulin resistant than peripheral ones, so free fatty acids are mobilized in greater concentrations from the visceral fat straight into the portal circulation, exposing the liver to high levels. It has been suggested that inflammatory cytokines produced by adipocytes also have a role in the aetiology of NASH. It might also be drug induced, by compounds such as methotrexate, amiodarone, warfarin, steroids and total parenteral nutrition, or by inborn errors of metabolism.

3.60 What is the treatment of NASH?

NASH responds extremely well to weight loss and increased physical activity, although extremely rapid weight loss, for instance after bariatric surgery, can temporarily exacerbate the situation because of increased lipolysis. In practice, the finding of abnormal liver function tests should be followed up more vigorously than previously thought, with serial blood tests and abdominal ultrasound, leading to referral where appropriate.

In many cases, NASH follows a benign clinical course and will only require monitoring, although weight loss in any case is beneficial. The effect of drug therapy on NASH has not been studied, although neither orlistat nor sibutramine is contraindicated. The use of metformin in non-diabetic patients with NASH is being studied because of the increase in insulin sensitivity induced by the drug.

SLEEP APNOEA

3.61 What is sleep apnoea?

Sleep apnoea (Pickwickian syndrome) is characterized by recurrent episodes of disrupted breathing, for 10 seconds or more, at a frequency of over 30 times per night, causing hypoxia and increased levels of carbon dioxide in the blood. It mainly disturbs the quality of rapid-eye-movement (REM) sleep and there can be as many as 20 or 30 episodes per hour; there is a strong association with snoring. The condition affects up to 4% of adults and is more common in men than women by about 4 to 1, although postmenopausal women who are not on HRT have an increased prevalence.

Spouses will often describe episodes when breathing stops for periods of up to a minute, followed by a loud grunt and the resumption of a normal pattern; sufferers describe startled awakening and choking. Daytime symptoms include drowsiness and somnolence, fatigue, memory loss, headaches and mood swings.

Studies show that almost half of patients complaining of daytime somnolence suffer from sleep apnoea (Coleman et al 1982). Complications include pulmonary hypertension, right heart failure, hypertension, stroke and cardiac arrhythmias, especially bradycardia, atrial flutter and ventricular tachycardia. The main cause of mortality is accidental death caused by falling asleep in inappropriate situations; there is a seven-fold increase in car accidents among sufferers of sleep apnoea. It is thought that there might be an increased risk of myocardial infarction but the evidence for this is inconclusive.

3.62 What is the link between obstructive sleep apnoea and obesity?

Obesity is the main risk factor for obstructive sleep apnoea, thought quite simply to be extra bulk of fatty tissue around the neck causing a degree of obstruction of the airways.

Most sufferers have a BMI >30 and men with a neck circumference of greater than 17 inches, or women greater than 16 inches, are at increased risk (Davies & Stradling 1990). It is likely that increased bulk of abdominal fat affects respiratory movements of the diaphragm and chest wall, especially in the supine position.

Central, rather than obstructive, sleep apnoea is a disorder of the respiratory centre in the brain and has no link with obesity.

3.63 How is sleep apnoea diagnosed and treated?

Sleep apnoea is diagnosed by performing overnight sleep studies (polysomnography).

The cornerstone of treatment is weight loss; a loss of 10% of body weight is associated with a 50% reduction in the severity of sleep apnoea. Sufferers should avoid coffee, cut down on alcoholic drinks and avoid sleeping pills, which might exacerbate apnoeic episodes. Patients who have difficulty losing weight will usually benefit from continuous positive airways pressure (CPAP), in which a mask is worn over the nose during sleep to force air, under pressure, through the nasal passages and overcome any airway obstruction.

Mechanical and dental devices used to manipulate the airway have limited success. Surgical procedures such as uvulopalatopharyngoplasty, which removes the bulk of the tissue from the back of the throat, have been shown to be of value in some patients but the considerable operative and postoperative risk, coupled with the uncertainty of success, make losing weight a far more desirable method.

PATIENT QUESTIONS

3.64 How does obesity affect pregnancy?

For a start, obesity makes it much more difficult to become pregnant because fatty tissue absorbs some of the hormones vital to pregnancy, putting them out of action. Fortunately, losing weight will correct the imbalance of hormones and increase the chance of conceiving. If a person manages to fall pregnant despite her weight problems, then obesity increases the chance of a problematic pregnancy. There is a greater risk of blood pressure and diabetes, a higher chance of pre-eclampsia and fits, and more likelihood of caesarian section and haemorrhage, which could even put the baby at risk. It is vital to combat any weight problems before trying to become pregnant to keep these risks as low as possible. Breast-feeding will reduce your baby's risk of obesity in later life, and will also help protect your own figure in the future.

3.65 Does obesity cause heart problems?

Obesity causes coronary heart disease and makes existing heart disease worse. It does this by causing high blood pressure and high levels of cholesterol and other fats in the blood, which clog up the arteries, leading to chest pain and often heart attacks. Obesity also causes the blood to be thicker and to clot more easily, which adds to the risk of both heart attacks and strokes. If you have heart disease, or if strokes and heart disease run in your family, you should look after your weight by eating sensibly and increasing you levels of physical activity, as well as by stopping smoking.

3.66 Is obesity linked to diabetes?

Yes, there is a very strong connection between diabetes and weight problems. An obese adult may be up to 100 times more likely to develop diabetes, and obese children are starting to suffer from the kind of diabetes that used to affect only old and middle-aged people. If you suffer from diabetes and have a weight problem you will find that by losing some weight your diabetes will be easier to control, and that your blood pressure and cholesterol will also improve considerably. If you are not diabetic, but other members of the family are, you should be extra careful to monitor your weight, otherwise you are likely to become diabetic yourself. If you are overweight and suffer from tiredness, fatigue, constant thirst and passing water all the time, you should get your blood sugar levels tested by your doctor.

3.67 What sorts of cancer are caused by obesity?

The main types linked to obesity are cancer of the large bowel, cancer of the breast and uterus in women, and cancer of the prostate in men. But there are also links with liver and kidney cancer, oesophageal and throat cancer, and lymphoma. The risk of cancer is reduced by losing weight. Obesity causes some cancers because the fatty tissue acts like a sponge and absorbs some of the body's natural sex hormones, leading to abnormalities in the breasts (especially after the menopause), the uterus and, in men, the prostate gland.

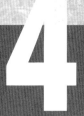

The psychological effects of obesity

4

4.1 Do overweight and obese people recognize their condition?

A MORI poll of overweight and obese people has found that, on the whole, most not only realize that they are overweight but also that weight is not merely a cosmetic issue but one that affects their health. The same poll revealed that 60% of overweight people admit that their health is affected by being overweight; 63% thought lack of exercise was the problem and 55% thought that a poor diet was a contributory factor.

4.2 Are fat people more jolly?

Circus 'fat folk' and freak show exhibits invariably had their name prefixed by the adjective 'jolly', whether or not they were in a particularly good mood at the time (*Fig. 4.1*).

However, when researchers at the University of Texas posed the question 'Are fat people more jolly?', they came up with an emphatic 'No!' (Roberts et al 2002). They analysed BMI, and studied eight indicators of mental health, including overall happiness, relationship satisfaction and optimism, and discovered that '…in no case did we observe better mental health among the obese. In sum, the obese were not more jolly'.

◀ **Fig. 4.1** In 1921, at age 18, 'Jolly Trixie' was with the Robinson Circus. Originally from Columbus, Ohio, she weighed 642 pounds.

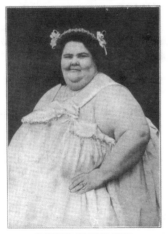

"JOLLY TRIXIE"

"WORLD'S FATTEST GIRL"
Weight 685 lbs. Age 21 yrs. Measuring: Hips, 92 inches; Bust, 84 inches; Thighs, 48 inches; Calfs 36 inches; Arms 34 inches. Wearing only a 4½ size shoe.
ON EXHIBITION WITH
The Chas. M. Abrahams' Greater Platform Shows
AND CONGRESS OF THE WORLD'S GREATEST
LIVING CURIOSITIES
TOURING THE WORLD.

4.3   How do overweight and obesity affect self-esteem?

A MORI survey (commissimed by Slimfast Foods Ltd and endorsed by the National Obesity Forum) in 2003 revealed that over 50% of overweight people lack self-confidence because of their weight, especially young women and most notably when swimming, exercising, on holiday or in pubs. In the same poll, 41% said they felt that they were judged more because of their weight than anything else and 25% had experienced insults from children. Obversely, 33% of the 'lean' population agree that they treat overweight people differently than others, and 25% believe that overweight people simply lack control. Dr Albert Stunkard, a foremost authority on depression and obesity, writing in his book *Pain of Obesity* (1980, p 75), quoted one of his patients describing herself as:

…a great mass of gray–green, amorphous material. Then at times I feel like a sloth. And just now, when I got up on the examining table, I felt like an elephant.

4.4   What is the association between obesity and depression?

It has long been accepted that there is a link between obesity and depression but there has never been any depth of evidence to absolutely define the connection. It is often unclear whether obesity or depression comes first in the cycle of weight gain and low self-esteem. Equally uncertain is the psychological effect of dieting: whether it is beneficial, by alleviating the stresses associated with obesity, or harmful, by accentuating anxieties and self-loathing when the almost inevitable rebound weight gain occurs.

One of the most famous men in eighteenth-century Britain was the physician Dr George Cheyne, who weighed 448 lbs at his peak and suffered from depression. He described his condition as:

…a *Disgust* or *Disrelish* of worldly *Amusements* and *Creature-Comforts*…tumultuous, overbearing *Hurricanes* in the Mind.

Various studies demonstrate the conflicting opinions. In the Swedish SOS study (Lindroos et al 1996), severely obese men and women displayed poor ratings for mental well-being, with increased depression and anxiety to a similar or greater degree than patients with metastatic malignant melanoma or tetraplegia. Wadden et al (1989), however, found that although overweight teenage girls were dissatisfied with their figure, they showed no signs of depression, although Rothschild et al (1989) found a positive association between obesity and depression in young adult males.

In an attempt to shed more light on the subject, an important study published in the *American Journal of Public Health* (Carpenter et al 2000) tested the relationship between body weight and clinical depression, suicide ideation and suicide attempts in more than 40 000 men and women. The study showed remarkable results. In women, obesity increased the risks of being diagnosed with major depression by 37% but in men obesity *decreased* this risk by 37%. A 10-unit increase in BMI increased the risk of suicide ideation and suicide attempts in women in the past year by 22%, whereas the risks were decreased by 26% and 55%, respectively, in men. In men, being underweight was associated with significantly higher risks of depression and suicide, although it is unclear whether the association was 'cause or effect' or whether, for instance, depressed men smoked more heavily, which might have had an effect on keeping weight down.

The conclusion was, therefore, that overweight women and underweight men are at higher risk of depression and suicide, and that the results were similar regardless of race.

4.5   What causes depression in obese patients?

No-one quite knows! It is tempting to assume that depression comes from extreme unhappiness at being fat, from disliking one's appearance in the mirror and from not being able to follow the same pursuits and exertions as leaner people, but it might not be as simple as that. It is thought that the cycle of dieting followed by weight gain followed by more dieting has a more profound depressant effect than merely being overweight or obese because of the added feelings of failure, whereas successful dieting has been shown to improve psychological function. To confuse matters further, some studies have suggested that low-calorie diets themselves have a specific association with depression.

Another possibility is that depression is a result of the attitude of others to the obese person. Social stigmata and penalties go hand in hand with obesity in a modern society that discriminates against fat people. This starts early in childhood when obese children are believed by their peers to be 'lazy, dirty, stupid, ugly, cheats and liars'. A Danish study showed that parental neglect is a strong predictor for obesity and it is not difficult to imagine how this could also lead to depression (Lissau & Sorensen 1994). A study of 10 000 Americans in 1981 showed that women with a BMI above the 95th centile achieved fewer years in school, were less likely to be married and had higher rates of household poverty than their leaner counterparts (Gortmaker et al 1993).

Others believe that obesity and depression go hand in hand because of the similar biochemical mechanisms between the two conditions, which both centre on the serotoninergic systems in the brain. Appetite suppressants such as fenfluramine increase levels of serotonin in the brain to reduce snacking and induce weight loss, and antidepressants such as fluoxetine inhibit the reuptake of serotonin, which can also lead to a degree of short-term weight loss. Sibutramine acts on both the serotoninergic and noradrenergic systems. This has led to a lot of supposition that the two conditions should be seen as different aspects of the same illness, and treated accordingly, but there is no convincing evidence to support this view.

A study from New York (Pine et al 2001) looked at children aged between 6 and 17 with major depression, and compared them with children with no psychiatric problems. When assessed 10 to 15 years later, those who were depressed as children had an average BMI of 26.1, compared with 24.2 in the control. Also, those who were depressed as children were twice as likely to be obese as adults.

A study in Minnesota (Ackard et al 2003) looked at 5000 middle- and high-school students and assessed the psychological effects of overeating. Seventeen per cent of girls and 8% of boys reported what they considered to be binge eating, but only 3% of girls and 1% of boys actually met the accepted criteria for binge eating disorder. Twenty-nine per cent of the girls who reported overeating, and 28% of boys, said they had tried to kill themselves, compared with only 10% of the rest of the group. The children who reported overeating did in fact have a tendency to overweight and obesity. This study not only measured the psychological implications of overweight and obesity but also gives some insight into obesity as a consequence of eating disorders.

4.6 What is the treatment for coexisting depression and obesity?

To successfully manage obesity in a depressed patient, the depression itself must be treated as a priority, by counselling or pharmacotherapy as appropriate, at the same time as traditional obesity management.

 It should also be borne in mind that lithium, as well as some antipsychotics, causes weight gain, and should be avoided if possible. Studies of SSRIs, in particular fluoxetine, demonstrate that they can induce weight loss early in treatment.

4.7 What are the psychological consequences of obesity?

Many studies show associations between obesity and psychological impairment. Although being obese is often perceived by members of the public as being indicative of greed, laziness, uncleanliness and unattractiveness, obese people are often mistaken for being 'jolly and plump'. Childhood obesity has also been associated with child neglect and in adulthood it is recognized, particularly among the morbidly obese, that childhood neglect and physical or sexual abuse often have a pivotal role in the development of disordered eating leading to obesity.

Obesity in adolescents and young adults has been shown to be associated with less successful education, reduced levels of income and increased psychological disturbance. In adolescence, the self-esteem of an obese child is diminished, more so in boys than in girls.

Prejudice is also commonly experienced in adult life, either directly as a result of negative attitudes from non-obese individuals, or indirectly, through an individual's feelings of decreased self worth and confidence.

The author has encountered patients who are afraid to lose weight for fear they may become more attractive and be at risk of sexual assault, a young woman who would sleep inside a sleeping bag under her duvet, to 'hide' from her partner because of self-loathing of her appearance, and countless individuals who have experienced loss of confidence because of unsolicited abuse when in public and, at times, private places. Conversely, weight loss can lead to marked improvements in self-esteem. One patient, having lost a significant amount of weight, finally attended her office Christmas party after 9 years of excuses because of her obesity. Other patients report increased perceptions of attractiveness, both subjective and objective, after weight loss, and a new-found confidence to go dancing, bowling or even simply to have a hair-cut. We should never underestimate the unseen psychological consequences of obesity.

4.8 Does obesity lead to psychological illness or does psychological illness lead to obesity?

The answer to both questions is probably 'yes'. There is no definitive research available but studies have shown associations between obesity and the development of psychological impairment, depressive illness and anxiety. In the Swedish Obese Subjects Study (Lindroos et al 1996), which looked at very obese patients undergoing bariatric surgery, the obese had a four-fold risk of anxiety and a seven-fold risk of depression. Similarly, other studies have shown associations between obesity and lower self-esteem. Some studies were unable to show any significantly impaired psychological health in their 18- to 23-year-old female group, but among women aged 45–49 there were significantly increased psychological problems, which increased further when the very heaviest obese were assessed separately. Clinical experience supports some available data that as many as 30% of morbidly obese patients attending a specialist obesity clinic report some form of disordered eating or frank eating disorder. It would seem likely that poor self-esteem, poor parenting, social deprivation and eating disorders contribute greatly to an individual's predisposition towards obesity in childhood and adult life.

4.9 What is emotional eating?

Many people describe comfort eating at times of stress, pressure or negative emotional state. This amounts to eating without relying on the usual stimulus of hunger to tell people when food is required. It has long been considered that this behaviour dates back to childhood, and even to breast-feeding, when eating and comfort were closely associated. Others admit to 'bingeing' on crisps or chocolates – common sense tells them to stop eating but they are powerless to resist until the box or packet is empty. It could be that these phenomena are due to the fact that there are common pathways in the brain between satiety and mood, as discussed above, and clearly the underlying stress or depression needs to be confronted for weight loss to be successful.

4.10 What is binge eating disorder?

Binge eating disorder (BED) is a specific, well-recognized eating disorder in its own right. Patients suffering from BED display the features of bulimia nervosa but without the purging, abnormal exercise regimes or other compensatory weight-loss-inducing features. The condition was recognized (but largely ignored) in 1959 but has recently been given greater importance. Its features are outlined in *Box 4.1*.

Studies suggest that 2.5% of adult women and 1.1% of men suffer from BED, of whom most but not all are obese (Spitzer et al 1993). The prevalence among patients attending obesity clinics is 20–30%, which emphasizes the importance of recognizing the condition without delay.

The treatment of BED is weight management using the conventional methods of dietary and lifestyle change as first-line treatment but with the addition of cognitive behavioural therapy (CBT). Strict diet regimes should be avoided because they are likely to aggravate the condition. CBT has been shown to be beneficial in patients with BED and without using it to help

---

BOX 4.1 Features of binge eating disorder

- Recurrent episodes of eating objectively large amounts of food within a discrete period of time accompanied by a subjective sense of lack of control during each episode
- The episodes are associated with three or more of the following: eating much more rapidly than normal; eating until feeling uncomfortably full; eating large amounts of food when not feeling physically hungry; eating alone because of being embarrassed by how much one is eating; feeling disgusted with oneself; feeling depressed or very guilty after overeating
- Marked distress about the binge eating behaviour
- The binge eating occurs, on average, at least 2 days a week for 6 months
- The binge eating is not associated with the regular use of inappropriate compensatory behaviours (e.g. purging, fasting, excessive exercise)

patients develop normal patterns and regain control of eating, weight management is unlikely to succeed. Depression and personality disorders have been linked with BED but it is unclear whether the abnormal eating pattern predates the emotional disorder or vice versa.

Dr Albert Stunkard (1980) has described the patient who first made him consider the existence of BED in the 1950s – a man named Hyman Cohen:

Everything seemed to go blank. I just said 'what the Hell' and started eating.' He started with cake, pieces of pie and cookies, then set out on a furtive round of the local restaurants, then went to a delicatessen, bought another $20 of food '...until my gut ached. I'll drink beer, maybe six or eight bottles to keep me going, then I'll want more food. I don't feel in control any more. I feel like Hell. I should be punished for the shameful act I've performed.'

4.11 What is night eating syndrome?

Like BED, night eating syndrome (NES) was recognized in the 1950s, by Albert Stunkard, as an abnormal eating pattern that was also associated with psychological and emotional factors. Sufferers are reported to be moody, tense, anxious, nervous and depressed; NES is thought to be associated with abnormal reactions to stress. Studies have shown changes in the circadian rhythm, with a disruption of the hypothalamopituitary axis. A study in February 2002 looked at the rise in stress hormones in response to the stimulus of corticotrophin-releasing hormone and found that NES sufferers had a weakened reaction compared with the control group (Birketvedt et al 2002).

Symptoms and criteria for NES are outlined in *Box 4.2*.

The prevalence of NES in the UK population is around 1–2%, rising to 10% of obese patients, and as many as 25% of grossly obese people. It is

---

BOX 4.2 Features of night eating syndrome

■ Morning anorexia, i.e. no appetite for breakfast; the first food of the day is delayed by several hours
■ Evening hyperphagia, i.e. excess food in the evening; 50% of the day's intake is eaten after the end of the evening meal and after 7 o'clock
■ The pattern has persisted for at least 2 months
■ Guilt feelings while eating. Eating causes tension and anxiety, not enjoyment
■ Frequent waking during the night, usually with eating during waking intervals
■ Mainly carbohydrates and sugars are eaten at inappropriate times
■ Involves continuous eating during the evening, unlike BED, in which eating is in short episodes

associated with obstructive sleep apnoea and restless leg syndrome, but has no association with nocturnal sleep-related eating disorder, which is more of a sleep disorder than an eating disorder and is characterized by eating during sleep, rather like sleep walking. A study of NES sufferers (Schenck & Mahowald 1994) emphasized the lack of hunger prior to the episodes of night eating, the 'automaticity' of the behaviour during waking intervals and varying levels of consciousness during eating. Most sufferers are said to have eaten fast and carelessly, with 30% having injured themselves! Treatment is predominantly behavioural rather than dietary, initially by persuading sufferers to have an early, substantial breakfast and to regain a normal eating pattern. The circadian rhythm should be reinforced by the appropriate amount of exercise during the day, with normal regular mealtimes and daily routines.

4.12 Does food addiction exist?

Opinions vary about whether food addiction is a genuine phenomenon or whether it is a product of the combination of external cues that make food seem irresistible. Those who say food addiction is *not* a genuine addiction point to the fact that, unlike cigarettes and drugs of addiction, food is a normal, essential part of life. They say that the concept of 'addiction' is merely a way of explaining the craving for certain foods and the lack of self-control needed to stop eating a food that one finds enjoyable. Hunger is a powerful sensation, and eating is a rewarding experience, and the combination of the two, especially when combined with the sight and smell of delicious food, could easily resemble true addiction.

However, there has been considerable research into the possible mechanisms of food addiction, in particular as to which chemical pathways might be responsible. Sufferers from seasonal affective disorder (SAD) lack sunlight-mediated serotonin, which not only causes them to be depressed but also seems to cause them to eat more during depressive episodes, especially carbohydrate-rich foods. It has been suggested that this is because carbohydrate metabolism leads to the formation of tryptophan, a precursor of serotonin, and that serotonin acts in the same way on the brain as SSRI antidepressants and is therefore the agent responsible for addiction.

Chocolate has been studied more than any foodstuff for signs of addictiveness and possible mechanisms, and although all sorts of attractive theories about caffeine, theobromine, phenylethylamine and tyramine have been proposed, it is probable that craving for chocolate is merely for the sensory experience.

Others have postulated that endogenous opioids are to blame, and a recent study (Volkow et al 2002) suggested dopamine – the 'pleasure chemical' – as a possible culprit. Subjects were allowed to see and smell their favourite food and, even without the pleasurable experience of tasting it, levels of dopamine in the brain were raised. This led investigators to believe that people eat for more reasons than just the pleasure of eating. Although the subject of food addiction is beloved of the tabloid press, the jury is still out on whether it is genuine.

4.13 Is there a link between obesity and Alzheimer's disease?

A small study (Galasko 2003) in Seattle suggests that high circulating levels of insulin increase the amount of amyloid, which, when laid down in the brain, is pathognomonic of Alzheimer's disease. The metabolic syndrome is characterized by hyperinsulinaemia, implying that there might be a link.

4.14 Is there a link between obesity and blindness?

A report in the *Archives of Ophthalmology* (Seddon et al 2003) links obesity to age-related macular degeneration, which is the leading cause of blindness in the US. Individuals with a BMI >30 have a 2.4-fold increased risk of progressing to advanced macular degeneration; physical activity tends to decrease the risk.

4.15 What is pseudotumour cerebri?

Pseudotumour cerebri (PTC) is a condition in which raised intracranial pressure occurs, with normal scans and investigations. Symptoms and signs include headache, diplopia, tinnitus, dizziness, nausea, vomiting, visual problems (occasionally blindness) and papilloedema, but with mental alertness. By far the most common cause of PTC is obesity, which is present in 66% of men with the condition and in up to 90% of women. PTC is more prevalent in women than men, in particular during childbearing years and in those more than 20% overweight. It is thought that obesity might cause a rise in abdominal, pleural and central venous pressure, which ultimately reduces drainage of cerebrospinal fluid (CSF) and increased intracranial pressure. Another theory relates to the peripheral conversion of androgens to oestrogens in adipocytes (*see* Q *3.44*), which might stimulate production of excess CSF. Many different surgical and pharmaceutical remedies for PTC have been attempted, but as long ago as 1958 weight loss was recognized to be the ideal treatment for the condition, although the degree of weight loss for resolution has never been accurately studied. Johnson et al (1999) recommended tried and tested weight-loss regimes, including goals of 5–10% weight loss, reduced fat intake and dietitian referral for an intake of approximately 1200 kcal, but occasionally used a blunter approach '…indicating that "the harsh reality is that it is your choice – 30 minutes exercise daily or risk permanent blindness".'.

4.16 Is there a stigma attached to being obese?

Social stigmata and penalties go hand in hand with obesity in a modern society that discriminates against fat people.

The 'personal view' section of the *British Medical Journal* explored the prejudices surrounding obesity in an article entitled 'Mangia meno' (Eat less; Dunea 1997):

Such gross obesity remains the butt of jokes and object of discrimination. Fat people remain 'the last persons you can safely kick about'; the 'last safe prejudice', even though in the early 1990s a [US] government agency declared obesity a protected category under the Federal Disabilities Act. But attitudes remain deeply ingrained. Last May, when a 500-lb Chicago woman died suddenly while taking a shower, police allegedly dragged her body by the feet and left it exposed, even jokingly telling the neighborhood urchins that they could take a peep for $5, leading to an official investigation for misconduct and a demonstration by 40 indignant neighbors carrying placards against the police.

 PATIENT QUESTIONS

4.17 Does obesity cause depression?

There is a definite link between obesity and depression, especially in women, but it is difficult to say whether the obesity causes the depression or if depression leads to comfort eating, lack of physical activity and therefore obesity. It certainly seems that yo-yo dieting could be a trigger for depression because of the repeated failure to lose weight in the long term. If a person suffers from a weight problem and also gets severe mood swings, tearfulness, insomnia and other signs of depression, it is important that these are addressed as part of the weight-management process, for instance by counselling or sometimes medication.

The costs of obesity

5

PQ PATIENT QUESTIONS

5.1 How are costs attributed to obesity?

Health economists have tried to calculate the financial implications of obesity, both to an individual and to the state. Costs are calculated by identifying the impact of obesity on comorbidities, and the resulting financial impact of providing medical treatment for those comorbidities. The majority of studies into the cost of obesity have been 'cost of illness' studies. These estimate the cost impact on the community and might look specifically at costs to a nation, an employer or healthcare provider. They are useful in providing information to guide health provision policies, to allow comparisons between different and even competing health problems, and to assess the magnitude of the effect of a specific disease on a societal basis. In calculating the costs of obesity, they must be categorized as *direct*, *indirect* and *intangible* costs.

5.2 What are the direct costs of obesity?

The direct costs of obesity attempt to calculate the costs of preventing, diagnosing and treating the comorbidities of the disease, and would most usually include the costs of treating cardiovascular disease, diabetes mellitus, hypertension and dyslipidaemia attributable directly to obesity. Different nations have calculated their own costs using varying criteria, and have included differing comorbid diseases, and so the statistics are not always directly comparable. What does seem reasonably consistent, however, is that the direct costs of obesity seem to account for between 2 and 6 % of national health expenditure. Such costs are assessed by evaluating cost attributed to medical time, both primary and secondary care, prescription costs, ambulance transportation and even such mundane items as heating, lighting and building maintenance. In the UK, estimates of direct costs were published by the National Audit Office in 2001, which calculated that £500 million was spent during 1998 treating obesity-associated disease in England. This would now seem to be a very conservative estimate. More recent figures for Scotland were published in 2003. With only one tenth of the population of England but comparable levels of obesity, direct costs of around £50 million would have been expected. In fact, Andrew Walker of Glasgow University (Walker, 2003) calculated the direct costs in Scotland to be £171 million, nearly four times higher than expected. Increased costs in Scotland might be attributed in part to simple inflationary rises over time, better recognition of obesity comorbid disease, and increased usage of NHS resources amongst the Scottish people. The implications for state healthcare providers are immense, as these figures can – under current circumstances – only continue to increase both in absolute terms and also as a rising percentage of NHS total expenditure. Only 2% of total direct costs are thought to be due to obesity management *per se*.

5.3   What are the indirect costs of obesity?

The indirect costs can be calculated by assessing the effects of obesity in contributing towards lost productivity at work, through impaired capability, increased tendency to sick days, poorer performance, earlier pensionable retirement and reduced total earning potential. Additional costs would include mortality costs through premature death as a result of obesity-related disease. In 2001, the National Audit Office estimated the indirect costs of obesity in England to be around £2.1 billion. It included the costs incurred by industry and the state in coping with obesity comorbid disease-related sick days (18 million sick days per annum), 40 000 lost years of working life and an estimate that those dying of an obesity-related disease were dying 9 years too early. In the US, 27% of the national workforce has a BMI ≥29. As the prevalence of obesity rises, so too will the indirect costs. Indirect costs are by their nature imprecise and most authors would seem to have been fairly conservative in their calculations.

> Taking direct and indirect costs together, the sum of £2.6 billion for England alone would account for more than 5% of total NHS expenditure per annum.

5.4   What are the intangible costs of obesity?

By definition, intangible costs are unquantifiable by financial models. They are, however, no less costly to suffering individuals. It is hard to put a price on the loss of self-esteem and confidence that can be experienced by an obese person (*see Chapter 4*) or on the effect of relationship difficulties and physical limitations encountered. It is difficult to evaluate the suffering of an obese person who cannot get to sleep because of depressive illness, and who wakes in the early hours from the pain of osteoarthritis in weight-bearing joints. It is impossible to truly determine the cost incurred by an individual experiencing prejudice from family, friends, medical and nursing staff, and even complete strangers.

Obesity is also associated with a decreased willingness of the individual to participate in social activities. In the Swedish Obese Subjects Study the majority of obese women described a reluctance to take a holiday away from home, buy clothes or attend the public swimming baths. In my practice I have encountered a 55-year-old man who agreed to exercise more but only after 9 p.m. – when it was dark – to avoid the cat-calls of the teenagers loitering the street. I have counselled a 40-year-old woman who, when walking along a street heard a car slow down beside her, saw the window being wound down and was greeted with 'get off the street you fat cow' and I have dealt with a 34-year-old woman who, after suffering her first stroke, with resultant dysphasia, was refused *any* inpatient investigation, her hospital notes recording: 'first stroke, morbidly obese, too big for CT scan, discharge to GP'! We cannot quantify the intangible costs but we cannot ignore them.

5.5 What is the social impact of obesity?

Obesity is not spread equally across the socioeconomic spectrum. Poor levels of nutrition and health awareness among lower socioeconomic groups result in a greater prevalence of overweight and obesity. High-fat, high-sugar food is often cheap and easy to prepare, and even simpler to reheat. The past few generations have seen a gradual decline in domestic culinary skills, and a greater dependency on 'convenience' foods.

At the same time, although levels of formal exercise participation in adults have increased over the past two decades, this is largely taking place in expensive sports centres and private gymnasiums, which are often not affordable by less well-off members of society.

As a result, obesity is much more prevalent among the lower socioeconomic groups. This in itself might perpetuate the cycle, as those who are obese are known to have less well paid jobs, have poorer opportunities for promotion, retire earlier, have higher personal health care costs and retire with less net worth than their leaner counterparts.

Clear socioeconomic differences have been shown to exist in preschool children. Preschool children from lower socioeconomic group households were more likely to eat high-fat foods such as burgers and kebabs, high-fat margarine, chips, sugars and tea. The same children were less likely to eat rice and wholemeal bread, high-fibre breakfast cereals, polyunsaturated margarine, cheese and fromage frais, oily fish, uncoated chicken, raw carrots and fruit and fruit juices.

5.6 Does obesity lead to health inequalities?

Obesity is one of the great unmet health inequalities. Predisposition to obesity is increased by lower socioeconomic status.

Middle-class individuals are far more likely to be interested in healthy nutrition, consume five portions of fruit and vegetables daily and provide healthy food choices for their families than people in lower social classes. They are also more likely to make time for structured formal exercise and to be able to afford a subscription to the local gym or tennis club. They probably have a car and shop at major supermarkets, where good-quality fresh food is available at competitive prices.

People in lower socioeconomic classes are less aware of nutritional health, less likely to have a car (and therefore less likely to shop at a supermarket), can ill-afford local shop prices and might have to rely on public transport to get the weekly shopping. Their children are more likely to go to a school where nutrition is not at the top of an already overcrowded agenda. They are more likely to buy cheaper, high-fat, high-sugar foods, simply because they can afford them. The local area may be less conducive to safe outdoor play and a greater reliance on TV for home entertainment results in diminished opportunity for physical activity. As a consequence, the prevalence of obesity is higher in this group. Morbidity and disability are more likely, average income is lower, opportunities are fewer and earlier retirement through ill health is more common, and thus the cycle is, to some degree, perpetuated.

Access to help to counter weight gain might also be more difficult for some social groups. Individuals in poorer communities are less likely to be able to afford to self-pay through a commercial weight-loss programme and are less likely to access web-based programmes. Inner-city healthcare providers might be too preoccupied in dealing with more obvious social issues, for example drug abuse and teenage pregnancy, to have the time and resources to fund and deliver weight-management services to those who are in need. Equally, medical practices might be reluctant to offer weight management for fear of opening a 'Pandora's box' of morbidity, and face soaring drug costs once they concede the need for weight management in their patients, who have a higher obesity prevalence to start with.

Although the prevalence of overweight and obesity in men is similar to women, men are less likely to seek advice on weight management from commercial agencies or medical services. Only 1% of clients registering with major weight-loss companies are male, and men account for only 20% of patients attending medical weight-management clinics in both primary and secondary care. This might be because men are less aware of weight as a health issue, or because of a reluctance on the part of men to seek professional advice, but attention must be given to the way in which weight-management services are delivered within the NHS. Weight-management clinics held during work times make it difficult for working men (and women) to attend, and men might feel embarrassed to attend during general medical clinics. The commercial sector has been modelled in a very female-oriented way, with little provision for male preference or needs. Some of the most successful men-oriented weight-management services have been based in barber-shops, at motor-cycle events or are internet based (see, for example, http://www.fatmanslim.com).

5.7 Would treating obesity save money in the long term?

Attempts have been made to create models to look at the possible cost savings if obesity were to be treated effectively and if weight loss was maintained long term. The majority of studies done on obesity treatment have been short term, with some as short as 12 weeks. Six to twelve months is the norm but some studies have extended up to and beyond 5 years, and these provide more convincing data. Many models use short-term clinical studies and then, making specific assumptions, predict long-term outcomes.

Jung (1997) predicted very significant decreases in morbidity and mortality in patients who lost just 10% of their body weight (*see Boxes 3.2 and 10.1*). Subsequent studies have not improved on these figures but many have predicted less enthusiastically on long-term disease risk. Oster et al. (1999) compared the relationship between BMI and the risks and costs of hypertension, stroke, dyslipidaemia, type 2 diabetes and ischaemic heart disease. They calculated that the effects of a sustained 10% weight loss would decrease expected medical care costs over a lifetime by up to US $5200. Compared to other chronic disease management costs these figures are impressive, as most chronic disease management results in extra costs, not cost reduction.

In the UK, the National Institute of Clinical Excellence (NICE) has looked at the effectiveness of orlistat and sibutramine in treating obesity. The number of quality added life years (QALYs) achieved by treating obesity with these medications were assessed. It is usual to assume that any cost-effectiveness ratio should be £35 000 or less to be considered as a cost effective solution. NICE calculated the cost of sibutramine treatment to be between £15 000 and £30 000 per QALY, and the cost of orlistat to be £20 000 to £30 000 per QALY. It would therefore seem reasonable to assume that obesity management is cost-efficient, although it has not yet been demonstrated to result in real cost savings.

5.8 Should the state fund obesity treatment?

Yes. The evidence of the effects of obesity, the huge financial and personal costs, the impact it has on personal and national economies, the benefits of modest sustained weight loss and the cost-effectiveness of treatment make a powerful argument for the NHS in the UK and health services elsewhere to implement and fund weight management.

Treatment of obesity can be shown to be effective in terms of weight loss, disease modification and cost effectiveness. The NHS has approved the provision of weight management, it remains for individual practitioners and healthcare organizations to make provision, both in terms of resources and training, to facilitate weight management in a state-run healthcare system. This does not in any way negate the concepts of individual and personal responsibility or the need for the state to promote obesity prevention on a national scale, but when presented with an obese patient, with or without comorbid disease, treatment can, and should, be made available.

5.9   What will happen to the NHS if the costs of obesity continue to rise?

At the moment, the costs of obesity in most developed nations account for between 2 and 5% of national health service expenditure but with the continuing rise in prevalence rates, costs are inevitably going to rise sharply. In nations where healthcare is government funded this raises serious concerns about the future of healthcare funding. For example, as a consequence of obesity it is estimated that the number of type 2 diabetics in the UK will double from 1.5 to 3 million in the next 10 years. This, and the other comorbid diseases of obesity, will cause a huge strain on NHS resources, both financial and logistical. This fact is not lost on governments across the world and much is being done to look for ways to minimize the crisis. The great difficulty is that any measures taken now will take years to show any tangible benefit, and so obtaining political support is not proving easy. However, unless quite radical changes are introduced soon, it may be too late and we may soon find healthcare provision in general being jeopardized by the overall cost of obesity.

 PATIENT QUESTIONS

5.10   Why does my doctor say he won't prescribe me weight loss medication as it's too expensive?

Weight loss medication isn't cheap, but used in the right patients its cost is far outweighed by the costs of obesity. Some doctors, concerned about their prescribing budgets, and maybe not fully understanding the seriousness of obesity, seem reluctant to offer even weight loss advice, let alone prescribe medication. Although it's difficult to quantify, available evidence would suggest that treating obesity may actually save the health service money. This is because the costs of treating resultant diabetes and heart disease, not to mention the cost of greater reliance on state benefits as a result of obesity, are immense. Each doctor has to weigh up the risks of treatment (and that includes cost) against those of the disease. However, if you are motivated to change your lifestyle, and make weight loss a long-term objective, then if weight loss drugs are appropriate for you, your doctor should seriously consider using them. It would be difficult to show in any individual cases, but it would seem that the benefits greatly outweigh the financial costs.

PATIENT QUESTIONS

Management: lifestyle and behavioural therapy

6.1   Is dieting a new idea?

There is an argument that any diet, however bizarre or eccentric, will have the benefit of focusing people's minds on their food and calorific intake, providing the motivation and stimulus to succeed. Clearly some diets suit certain individuals and others don't. William Banting, Queen Victoria's Royal Undertaker to the Throne, was advised to lose weight because of his deteriorating hearing and vision; so successful was he in shedding the pounds that he published his story in his *Letter to the public on corpulency*; the world's first ever commercial diet. Foremost among Mr Banting's recommendations was seven units of alcohol per day; one can only guess at how people managed to stick to such a strict regime week after week without abandoning the system!

In the eighteenth century, Dr George Cheyne famously invented the lettuce diet, which would be utterly frowned upon today but which seems to have added many years to the good doctor's life.

History is littered with dietary manuals, hints and systems, and the likelihood is that today's dietary vogues and fashions will look equally ridiculous in 10 years time. Some early examples are given in *Box 6.1*.

BOX 6.1   Early examples of popular dietary advice

From the late eighteenth to the early twentieth centuries there were widely varying approaches to weight management (Gilman Thompson 1909):

- Epstein believed that fat should be allowed in the diet because, although high in calories, it promoted satiety. This is the opposite of what we now believe – fat is high in calories but poor at promoting satiety compared with protein or carbohydrate.
- Oertel recommended withholding fluid as a means of reducing fat, a regime attempted – apparently successfully – by Otto von Bismarck.
- It is no great surprise that the weight management scheme put forward by Weir Mitchell gained popular success. It comprised an intriguing combination of milk, shellfish, rest and Swedish massage.
- Yeo was very specific about precisely which alcoholic drink was preferable to induce maximum weight loss: Hock, Moselle or light claret, but certainly no beer or porter.
- This theme was continued by Dujardin, who shunned the evils of soup of all kinds, recommending wine as an alternative.

No publisher in the world would have wasted his ink to publicize such remedies unless there was popular interest and some money to be earned and, if people genuinely lost weight on such regimes, they should be given the appropriate credit.

DIET IN THE MANAGEMENT OF OBESITY

6.2 What are the fundamentals of dietary treatment for overweight and obese patients?

The basic rules of diet and nutrition are succinctly and coherently set out in the British Nutrition Foundation's concept 'the balance of good health' (*Fig. 6.1*). Dietary recommendations vary from the normal in certain conditions such as metabolic syndrome, but the concept is an excellent basis for dietary education.

6.3 What alternative advice is available?

There are countless commercial diets thrust upon the public in newspapers, bookshops, on TV, the internet and on the coffee morning circuit. Many of these may have benefits and others remarkable, or alarming, ramifications.

To succeed and make money for its inventor, any commercial diet must have a unique and novel aspect or idiosyncrasy that makes it different to those which have gone before. It is exactly this idiosyncrasy that should make us treat the diet with suspicion. There has been no great evolutionary advance in the human digestive or metabolic systems, or major

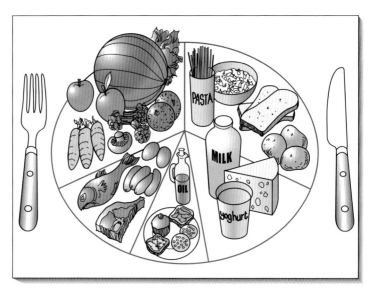

▲

Fig. 6.1 The balance of good health.

breakthrough in the science of nutrition, to necessitate brand new diet theories. On the contrary, new diets either repackage what we already know in different, easily understood words and phrases – which should be encouraged – or else are fad diets without scientific basis – which shouldn't. There is a growing body of opinion, especially in the US, known as the 'undieting' lobby, which takes the argument one step further and is opposed to any sort of structured diet programme. The National Eating Disorders Association in The US describes dieting as a dangerous eating disorder, defining it as:

Any attempt in the name of weight loss, 'healthy eating', or body sculpting to deny your body of the essential, well-balanced nutrients and calories it needs to function to its fullest capacity.

Its literature spells out the dangers of yo-yo dieting (including 'negative impacts on the metabolism'), psychological problems (including depression) and progression to other eating disorders. It reports that 40–50% of women in the US are dieting at any one time, 40–60% of high-school girls are dieting and that 46% of 9- to 11-year-olds are dieting 'sometimes or very often' (see http://www.nationaleatingdisorders.org).

Although extremely eloquently put and vigorously argued, these views are rather extremist and overlook the simple fact that reputable weight-loss diets save lives, particularly in the case of diabetics and sufferers of coronary heart disease.

A sensible approach is to treat 'dietary change' as one thing, by educating patients on good and bad nutrition and giving them the skills to permanently alter their own feeding habits, but to treat 'Diets' with caution. Patients have the ability to choose their preferred method of losing weight, be it through primary care or buying a book, attending a private slimming clinic or accessing help on the internet. Primary care has neither the time nor the resources to cope with each and every obese person without outside help.

Although today's commercial diets have a more scientific basis than those discussed in Q 6.1, there are still some slightly unusual concepts being promoted, which may not entirely fit in with what we learnt at medical school. It is part of the job of the primary care team to tiptoe through the minefield of the modern commercial diets and to encourage patients to follow a path that is not only clinically acceptable but also suits the individual's taste, social circumstances, working environment and family life.

6.4   Are commercial diets a good way of 'watching weight'?

Without doubt, commercial diets are the only way for some people to cope with the challenge of weight management. However, for others the goal is to develop for themselves the skills and the motivation to manage their diet and lifestyle in a manner that suits them. For these individuals it is essential to learn the basic rules of nutrition, and to be provided with the tools to decide for themselves what long-term strategy is appropriate (and to judge what combination of milk, lettuce, soup and alcohol is best for them!).

6.5 What are the cornerstones of dietary education?

Certain basic nutritional guidelines will equip patients to choose their own diet and calorific intake. There are also very many facts and figures on display in books and on supermarket shelves; nutritional information shown in big brightly coloured letters on the front of packs of food and more sobering statistics in tiny letters hidden on the back. Such tricks are designed to confuse us and make us buy more food. It is important for us, when educating patients, to get the balance right; to give enough information to enable patients to make sensible, informed choices without making their heads spin with too many facts. The label on the back of most packaged foods contains a wealth of important information, whereas the brightly coloured logo on the front of a pack might contain some very misleading ideas. As obese people are going to have to watch their weight for the rest of their lives, they must know how to avoid the pitfalls devised by food manufacturing companies for unsuspecting customers in their local supermarket.

6.6 What is the Atkins diet?

The Atkins diet is essentially a low-carbohydrate, high-fat, high-protein diet. Dr Robert Atkins caused controversy, made headlines and aroused public interest up until his tragic death from a head injury in April 2003 aged 70. His revolutionary views caused feelings to run high among nutritionists, clinicians and most of all obese and overweight people the world over. His suggestion that carbohydrates should be reduced as part of dietary treatment for overweight and obesity is as old as the hills. In 1864, William Banting, in his *Letter on Corpulence* (*see* Q 6.1), told his followers to 'reduce farinaceous foods'. Foods such as bread, pasta, potatoes, cereals, sugars and fruits, and usually alcohol, are restricted in favour of protein and fat. The concept is that reduced carbohydrate lessens the burden on the body's insulin supplies, thus reducing insulin resistance. But the thought of having a deliberately high-fat diet, with lashings of butter, fried food and fatty meats, has set alarm bells ringing among the established medical hierarchy. The American Heart Association issued a position statement saying that high-fat diets would cause disruption of normal lipid metabolism, high triglycerides and LDL:

High-protein, low-carbohydrate diets put people at risk for heart disease. The saturated fat and cholesterol content of the diet will raise the bad cholesterol and increase the risk for cardiovascular disease, particularly heart attacks.

It pointed the finger particularly at people who stopped losing weight on the diet but continued the high-fat intake. But Dr Atkins disagreed, issuing a reply based on several recent studies indicating that high triglycerides and low HDL were linked to high carbohydrate diet, and that because of the increased bodily fat metabolism in his diet, the HDL:LDL ratio can improve significantly. His critics responded by saying that there is generally an improvement in lipid profile with weight loss but that it is still unhealthy to eat large quantities of saturated fat. The nutritionists for the Atkins diet do, however, recommend 'healthy fats' and encourage such foods as oily fish, as well as vitamin supplementation.

The American Dietetic Association publicly stated its concern about high levels of protein affecting the kidneys and liver; studies have also shown a link with renal colic (Costain 2003 p 204), but once again Dr Atkins denied the link.

Various experts have expressed their worries about the diet, saying that no long-term studies have been undertaken, primarily because of the recent rise to popularity of the system. The diet has been said to be physiologically unsustainable because the body becomes ketotic as a result of fat metabolism leading to acetone as the end product, which leads to raised pulse and respiration, as well as bad breath. But, once again, long-term evidence of these effects is lacking.

Another major criticism of the diet is that it is becoming increasingly clear that fruit and vegetables are protective of good health (and hence they are being promoted in schools and supermarkets), which leads to concern about the massive reduction of these foods in low-carbohydrate diets.

The main resistance to the Atkins diet, however, is the likelihood that weight loss will turn out to be only temporary. Carbohydrate, stored as glycogen in the liver, is bound with fluid. When this store is depleted, much of the weight lost is water, which is rapidly regained when a person finishes the Atkins plan and eats carbohydrate again. Weight maintenance after weight loss is therefore a potential problem for low carbohydrate devotees, although this is addressed in the plan.

Currently, it seems that there is no definitive answer as to whether or not low-carbohydrate diets are safe or effective; there appears to be evidence on both sides. However, it is certainly true that some patients do rapidly lose significant amounts of weight on the Atkins diet, and some appear to be able to maintain considerable weight loss. There is considerable scepticism and suspicion surrounding low-carbohydrate diets, and certainly no consensus as to their value in long-term weight management. They are undeniably popular but should be approached with caution.

6.7   What are the drawbacks of the Atkins diet?

Apart the reservations that many clinicians have about the diet, there are problems from the patient's perspective in sticking to the regime. It seems that the range of foods, and therefore tastes and flavours, is somewhat limited, leaving the dieter bored and unsatisfied, although never hungry. An unremitting, unlimited intake of steak after steak, bacon, sausage, egg, cheese, and so on can become monotonous without the variety introduced by carbohydrate, and does result in patients abandoning the regime for the sake of a piece of forbidden fruit! The diet lacks calcium and fibre, causes constipation and can be expensive.

6.8 There seem to be millions of diets out there; how do I know what's what?

Each commercial diet is unique in some way; each has its own individual feature that acts as its unique selling point. Low-carbohydrate diets have been with us for generations, some recommend high protein and others, like the Atkins, high fat. The following are different forms of restricted carbohydrate diet.

THE MONTIGNAC DIET

Founded on the premise that 'we should sweep away scruples and allow our epicurean instincts full rein', this diet is based on the glycaemic index (GI) of different carbohydrates and focuses on foods with a GI less than 50 (*Table 6.1*). The system, described in the book *I eat therefore I slim*, limits starches, sweets and alcohol strictly for an initial period, followed by a maintenance phase during which wine, cheese, chocolate and even foie gras are acceptable. The theory goes that foods with a high GI are absorbed rapidly into the bloodstream, stimulating overproduction of insulin and all the associated problems described in *Q 3.14*. 'Sugar should be labelled with a skull and crossbones' says Montignac, pointing out that high sugar and insulin levels lead to the laying down of body fat, so high GI foods (e.g. white bread and butter) should be avoided and certainly not mixed with fatty food.

The glycaemic index of different foods is undoubtedly important; low GI foods are a source of sustained, slow-release energy and are preferable to highly refined sugars, which appear in the bloodstream rapidly. The Montignac diet is less draconian than Atkins and allows the dieter to eat a more socially acceptable mixture.

Criticism of the diet is similar to that directed at the Atkins diet; weight loss is due entirely to calorie restriction and high fat is likely to lead to heart problems; there may also be a lack of calcium and other nutrients. Additionally, it has been said that the Montignac diet encourages too high an alcohol intake; the body has no mechanism to store alcohol so it takes priority as the first substance to be metabolized, leaving any fat eaten at the same time to be laid down as adipose tissue.

TABLE 6.1 Glycaemic index of a selection of popular foods

Food	Portion size	Glycaemic index (GI)	Carbohydrate (g) per portion	kcals per portion
High GI foods (GI = 60–100)				
Breakfast cereals				
Cornflakes	1 small bowl (30 g)	84	26	108
Rice Crispies	1 small bowl (30 g)	82	27	111
Cheerios	1 small bowl (30 g)	74	23	111
Shredded Wheat	2 (45 g)	67	31	146
Weetabix	2 (40 g)	69	30	141
Grains/pasta				
Couscous	5 tbsp (150 g)	65	77	341
Brown rice	6 tbsp (180 g)	76	58	254
White rice	6 tbsp (180 g)	87	56	248
Breads				
Bagel	1 (90 g)	72	46	241
Croissant	1 (60 g)	67	23	216
Baguette	3 inches long (40 g)	95	22	108
White bread	1 large slice (38 g)	70	18	85
Wholemeal bread	1 large slice (38 g)	69	16	82
Pizza	1 large slice (115 g)	60	38	288
Crackers and biscuits				
Puffed crispbread	1 slice (10 g)	81	7	32
Ryvita	1 slice (10 g)	69	7	32
Water biscuit	1 (8 g)	78	6	35
Rice cakes	1 (8 g)	85	6	28
Shortbread	1 (13 g)	64	8	65
Vegetables				
Parsnip	2 tbsp (65 g)	97	8	43
Baked potato	1 medium (180 g)	85	22	94
Boiled new potato	7 small (175 g)	62	27	116
Mashed potato	4 tbsp (180 g)	70	28	188
Chips	average (165 g)	75	59	450
Swede	2 tbsp (60 g)	72	1	7
Broad beans	2 tbsp (120 g)	79	7	58
Fruit				
Cantaloupe melon	1 slice (200 g)	65	6	26
Pineapple	1 slice (80 g)	66	8	33
Raisins	1 tbsp (30 g)	64	21	82
Watermelon	1 slice (200 g)	72	14	62

TABLE 6.1 Glycaemic index of a selection of popular foods—contd

Food	Portion size	Glycaemic index (GI)	Carbohydrate (g) per portion	kcals per portion
Dairy products				
Ice cream	1 scoop (60 g)	61	14	62
Drinks				
Fanta	375 mL can	68	51	191
Lucozade	250 mL bottle	95	40	150
Isostar	250 mL can	70	18	68
Gatorade	250 mL bottle	78	15	56
Squash (diluted)	250 mL glass	66	14	54
Snacks and sweets				
Tortilla/corn chips	1 bag (50 g)	72	30	230
Mars bar	1 standard (65 g)	68	43	287
Muesli bar	1 (33 g)	61	20	154
Sugars				
Glucose	1 tsp (5 g)	100	5	19
Sucrose	1 tsp (5 g)	65	5	19
Maltodextrin	1 tsp (5 g)	105	5	19
Moderate GI foods (GI = 40–59)				
Breakfast cereals				
All Bran	1 small bowl (40 g)	42	19	104
Sultana Bran	1 small bowl (30 g)	52	20	91
Porridge (with water)	1 small bowl (160 g)	42	14	78
Muesli	1 small bowl (50 g)	56	34	183
Grains/pasta				
Buckwheat	4 tbsp (80 g)	54	68	292
Bulgar wheat	4 tbsp (56g)	48	44	196
Basmati rice	4 tbsp (60 g)	58	48	215
Noodles	4 tbsp 230 g cooked	46	30	143
Macaroni	4 tbsp 230 g cooked	45	43	198
Spaghetti	4 tbsp 220 g cooked	41	49	229
Breads				
Pitta bread	1 large (75 g)	57	43	199
Rye bread	1 slice (25 g)	41	11	55

TABLE 6.1 Glycaemic index of a selection of popular foods—
contd

Food	Portion size	Glycaemic index (GI)	Carbohydrate (g) per portion	kcals per portion
Biscuits and cakes				
Digestive	1 (15 g)	59	10	71
Oatmeal	1 (13g)	55	8	57
Rich Tea	1 (10 g)	55	8	40
Muffin	1 (68 g)	44	34	192
Sponge cake	1 slice (60 g)	46	39	181
Vegetables				
Carrots	2 tbsp (60 g)	49	3	14
Boiled potato	2 medium (175 g)	56	30	126
Peas	2 tbsp (70 g)	48	7	48
Sweetcorn	2 tbsp (85 g)	55	17	94
Sweet potato	1 medium (130 g)	54	27	109
Yam	1 medium (130 g)	51	43	173
Pulses				
Baked beans	1 small tin (205 g)	48	31	166
Fruit				
Apricots	1 (40 g)	57	3	12
Banana	1 (100 g)	55	23	95
Grapes	1 small bunch (100 g)	46	15	57
Kiwi	1 (68 g)	52	6	29
Mango	half (75 g)	55	11	43
Orange	1 (208 g)	44	12	54
Papaya	half (175 g)	58	12	47
Peach	1 (121 g)	42	8	36
Plum	1 (58 g)	39	5	20
Sultanas	1 tbsp (18 g)	56	12	50
Dairy products				
Custard	2 tbsp (120 g)	43	20	140
Drinks				
Apple juice	1 glass (160 mL)	40	16	61
Orange juice	1 glass (160 mL)	46	14	58
Snacks and sweets				
Crisps	1 packet (30 g)	54	16	159
Milk chocolate	1 bar (54 g)	49	31	281

TABLE 6.1 Glycaemic index of a selection of popular foods—contd

Food	Portion size	Glycaemic index (GI)	Carbohydrate (g) per portion	kcals per portion
Sugars				
Honey	1 heaped tsp (17 g)	58	13	49
Low GI foods (GI = 1–39)				
Pulses				
Butter beans	4 tbsp (120 g)	31	22	124
Chick peas	4 tbsp (140 g)	33	24	168
Red kidney beans	4 tbsp (120 g)	27	20	124
Green/brown lentils	4 tbsp (160 g)	30	28	164
Red lentils	4 tbsp (160 g)	26	28	160
Soya beans	4 tbsp (120 g)	18	6	169
Fruit				
Apples	1 (100 g)	38	12	47
Dried apricots	5 (40 g)	31	15	63
Cherries	1 small handful (100 g)	22	10	39
Grapefruit	half (80 g)	25	5	24
Peaches tinned	half tin (120 g)	30	12	47
Pear	1 (160 g)	38	16	64
Plum	1 (55 g)	39	5	20
Dairy products				
Full cream milk	half pint (300 mL)	27	14	198
Skimmed milk	half pint (300 mL)	32	15	99
Yoghurt (low fat fruit)	1 carton (150 g)	33	27	135
Snacks and sweets				
Peanuts	1 small handful (50 g)	14	4	301
Sugars				
Fructose	1 tsp (5 g)	23	5	19

THE SCARSDALE DIET

This diet (named after the place, not a person) had its place in the spotlight in the 1970s and is still used today despite the tragic death of its author – Dr Herman Tarnower – who was shot by his lover in 1980. It restricts intake to around 1000 calories, with reduced carbohydrate, low fat and high protein, and is limited to 2 weeks at a time, followed by a 'keep-trim' programme. It can cause dramatic weight loss because of the calorie reduction but isn't nutritionally balanced and generally results in rebound weight gain.

THE STILLMAN DIET

This diet is also only used for short-term 'plateau-breaking'. It comprises low carbohydrate, high protein and low fat, including as much lean meat, fish, shellfish and eggs as required, with high water, black tea and coffee intake.

THE PROTEIN POWER

This diet allows a modest, carefully monitored amount of carbohydrate intake each day in order, it is claimed, to closely control insulin production. It is high in protein and fat, and falls into a similar category to the Atkins diet.

THE ZONE DIET

This diet demands that 40% of calorie intake should be carbohydrate, 30% protein and 30% fat, and includes the use of Zone supplement bars. Rebound weight gain is considered to be the main problem. It also differentiates between 'good' and 'bad' carbohydrates, leading to a restriction in vegetable intake.

6.9 What are food-combining diets?

Confusingly, food-combining diets are based on the principle of separating different kinds of food. They work on the principle that eating different categories of food, for instance carbohydrate and protein together, interferes with digestion and should be avoided. Starchy food, the theory goes, requires alkaline conditions for digestion, whereas protein requires an acidic digestive medium. When eaten together, the pH becomes neutral, digestion is arrested, undigested food becomes a substrate for bacteria, which multiply and produce toxins which poison us. Although many clinicians claim that there is no scientific evidence to support this theory, these diets remain popular because, if followed diligently, they will cause moderate weight loss because of the reduction in calories consumed. The emphasis in these diets is on eating natural wholesome food and avoiding processed, high-fat, high-sugar meals. However, this also involves the dieter in a lot of time-consuming food preparation and cooking.

The first diet to teach food-combining theory was the Hay diet, formulated in the early twentieth century by William Hay, who allegedly cured himself of hypertension, heart and renal disease by practising what he preached, which was a 'natural wholefood diet with at least 50% fresh fruit, vegetables and salad'. Protein-based food such as meat and cheese should be taken at separate meals to carbohydrates such as pasta and potatoes. His diet has spawned an entire industry of related food-combining books, websites and TV celebrities.

6.10 What are detox diets?

Detox diets are designed to rid our systems of all the 'nasty' chemicals we encounter in day-to-day life, including pollution, drugs, crop sprays, processed foods, alcohol and so on. Even though we have a perfectly acceptable system involving the liver, kidneys and bowel to rid the body of such compounds, detox diets claim to get rid of the toxic overload while at the same time inducing weight loss. The typical detox diet contains organic fruit and vegetables, nuts, seeds and lots of mineral water in preference to sugars, processed, packaged and canned foods. Although there are sensible nutritional reasons to eat plenty of fruit and vegetables, and to have a moderate alcohol consumption, detox diets fail because they aren't sustainable or balanced, due to the lack of calcium and other vital nutrients, and because they don't educate patients the correct rules of diet and nutrition.

6.11 What are high-fibre diets?

High-fibre diets, such as the F-plan diet of the 1980s, teach dieters to increase their fibre intake, increasing bulk, which in theory causes early satiety with less energy consumed. This means that low-energy-dense foods displace high-energy-dense foods from the diet. It also has the effect of increasing intake of fruit and vegetables, in line with recommendations, and reducing fat, although sometimes causing bowel dysfunction.

6.12 What are very-low-calorie diets?

Very-low-calorie diets (VLCDs) are extreme forms of weight loss diets, also known as modified fasts. They are formula diets, usually in liquid form, and provide a calorific intake of between 400 and 800 kcal per day, as well as being balanced and nutritionally complete. Initial weight loss can be expected to be high, often around 6 lb per week. They are not suitable for the average dieter, who needs to lose weight for cosmetic purposes, or to fit their bathing costume, or even for the moderately obese patient who needs to lose weight for medical reasons. Such patients should lose weight by reverting to a normal healthy balanced diet, combined with activity and lifestyle changes to maintain a healthy weight.

VLCDs, by their very nature, are for short-term use, and only in exceptional circumstances and under supervision. They were introduced in the 1970s as a means of rapid weight loss but were beset with safety problems relating to the loss of lean body mass as well as fatty tissue that occurs with such rapid weight loss. In the UK, the Committee on Medical Aspects of Food Policy (COMA) produced a report in 1987 indicating what the content of these formula diets should be, including minimum calories and protein levels, and limiting their use to individuals with BMI >30, under close supervision. In The US the National Task Force for Prevention and Treatment of Obesity (1993) defines VLCDs as having less than 800 kcal. The COMA report limited the duration of such diets to 4 weeks but in practice the initial 400-kcal phase is often followed by a longer period in which 'normal' food is added to the formula diet.

Various studies have been done to demonstrate the effects of VLCDs on obesity and its comorbidities. Capstick et al (1997) showed that they produced substantial weight loss in obese individuals with type 2 diabetes, and a subsequent improvement in glycaemic control. Saris (2001) concluded that VLCD with active follow-up was related to long-term weight maintenance success. As with any modality of treatment, VLCDs are most successful when used in conjunction with other types of treatment.

6.13 What is a low-calorie diet?

A low-calorie diet (LCD) is another example of formula food but differs in some ways from a VLCD. Once calorie intake falls below 1200 kcal, it is impossible to keep a correct nutritional balance by eating 'normal' food alone, so LCD formulae provide some calories and nutrients that, when added to a restricted 'normal food' diet, maintain the overall balance. As VLCDs make up the whole daily intake of calories, vitamins, minerals and so on, they must be nutritionally complete in their own right.

6.14 What is a milk diet?

A milk diet is similar to a VLCD except the 'formula' is 1.5–2 L cows milk combined with vitamins and iron, providing over 800 kcal per day. Garrow et al (1989) compared the milk diet with a VLCD, and found no significant difference in weight loss. Many people cannot tolerate so much milk and compliance is often poor.

6.15 What are meal replacements?

Meal replacements are nutritionally balanced formula foods in the form of shakes, soups or bars, which are designed to replace one or two main meals a day. The substitute usually contains 200–400 kcal. The remainder of the day's intake – the third meal plus any snacks – comprises food carefully selected by the consumer guided by the educational and supportive material supplied as part of the meal replacement 'plan'. Ditschuneit et al (1999) studied the effects of one or two meal replacements on body weight and biomarkers of disease risk, compared to a control group who took a traditional weight-loss diet and observed the long-term benefits for 4 years. Not only did they find a weight loss of 11% in the meal replacement group compared with 8% in the control group, but there were also improvements in blood pressure (−11%) triglycerides (−37%) glucose (−11%) and insulin. Writing in the *European Journal of Clinical Nutrition*, the same team reported the improvement in dyslipidaemia after 4 years, including a reduction of 14.7% total cholesterol and a 6.6% reduction in LDL (Ditschuneit et al 2002).

6.16 What are single-food diets?

Diets such as the grapefruit diet or the cabbage soup diet are based on the premise that certain foods have fat-burning properties. There is no evidence to support these claims; weight loss can be dramatic but only because of the strict calorie reduction involved. The cabbage soup diet is generally a 7-day, quick-fix diet comprising vast quantities of homemade cabbage soup supplemented by vegetables, rice and occasional meat.

The New Beverley Hills diet allows only fruit, and not only that, but different fruits should not be consumed on the same day; some days only melon should be eaten, on other days grapes. A diet consisting exclusively of fruit has the obvious drawbacks of being tedious and of containing insufficient fat, protein, iron, calcium, vitamin B_{12} and many other vital nutrients.

6.17 Which diet is best?

Dietary treatment is fundamental to the management of obesity, but unless the obese person is willing and able to make long-term changes in lifestyle (of which diet is the most important aspect) treatment will fail. However merely 'going on a diet' for a finite period may cause temporary weight loss, but this weight will be regained when the 'diet' is abandoned (Garrow 1999).

The best diet is the one that provides the patient with the necessary support, skills and knowledge to permanently address the deficiencies in his or her consumption of food that helped cause the obesity in the first place.

The most appropriate 'diet', and the most likely to result in long-term weight loss is a low-fat diet, rich in complex carbohydrates and well balanced with protein, and other nutrients. The expression 'balance of good health' (*see Fig 6.1*) has been coined to describe – concisely and attractively – how to achieve this standard.

6.18 What is a low-fat, high-carbohydrate diet?

A high-carbohydrate diet is the one that adheres most closely to current nutritional recommendations and therefore is the form of diet most often used by slimming agencies such as Slimming World, Weight Watchers and Rosemary Conley. Slimming groups such as these provide on-going support, advice and motivation on lifestyle and physical activity as well as teaching food and nutrition skills, and are extremely useful in providing support and camaraderie to people attempting to lose weight. Overweight and obese men are traditionally apprehensive about, and reluctant to attend, slimming clinics, and are notoriously hopeless at turning up to see their GP. Fat Man Slim is an internet-based behavioural change programme for men designed to overcome such barriers (see www.fatmanslim.com).

LIFESTYLE AND EXERCISE

6.19 What is the importance of physical exercise in the management of obesity?

Increased physical activity is vital in the management of obesity. Professor Kenneth Fox, one of the foremost authorities explains:

The human body has evolved to accommodate vigorous physical activity, and inactivity can be regarded as the abnormal, rather than normal. It should not, therefore, be surprising that inactivity is associated with ill health (British Nutrition Foundation 1999).

Weight gain occurs when the number of calories ingested is greater than the number of calories being burnt off. The combination of the modern diet (with its propensity for high-calorie, energy-dense food) and increasing sedentary behaviour is therefore a potent obesogenic one.

The Pima Indians of Southern Arizona (see Q 1.12) are a dramatic illustration of changing lifestyle having a catastrophic effect on weight and health. For 30 000 years the Pima Indians were lean, fit, hunter-gatherers and farmers. But in the 1930s they gained greater access to 'Western' sedentary lifestyles and they are now the 'fattest people on Earth' and have appalling health problems resulting from their obesity.

Just as the Pima Indians' original day-to-day life included physical activity, so did the day-to-day life of most Americans and Europeans. In 1735, John Arbuthnot wrote:

The most common cause of fat is too great a Quantity of Food, and too small a Quantity of Motion, in plain English Gluttony and Laziness. You may see in an Army forty thousand Foot-Soldiers without a fat man amongst them.

Apart from a career as a foot soldier, many other occupations were physical or manual: farming, mining, industry and so on. In the twenty-first century our employment has become more sedentary: we drive to and from work, or use public transport; we sit all day at computers or on the telephone and we use energy-saving devices such as automatic doors and escalators. Our leisure time is also increasingly sedentary; more and more people have one or more computers at home, so we can work on one machine while the children play games on another. Similarly, TVs and DVDs are becoming more common and TV viewing times increase with the number of channels available. Not all of us have high-tech, office-based jobs but we have all reduced our level of physical exertion because of modern life, whether it is using the lift instead of the stairs, using the remote control instead of getting up and changing the TV channel or using mobile phones instead of jumping out of our chair to answer the telephone and, while we're there, ordering a take-away instead of cooking (*Fig. 6.2*).

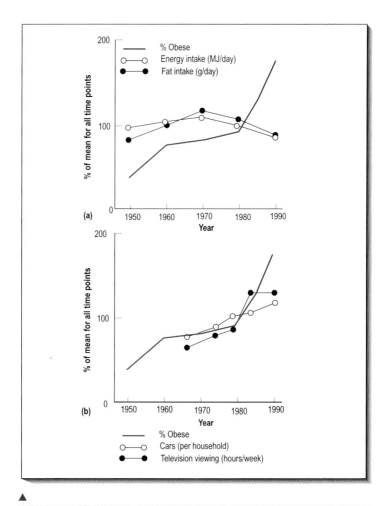

Fig. 6.2 (a) Trends in dietary intake and (b) in inactivity indicators in relationship to obesity in the UK. The values show percentages from each time point based on an average of 1000% timespan (from Prentice and Jebb 1995, with permission from the BMJ Publishing Group).

6.20 How important is physical activity in weight management?

Physical activity is helpful in losing weight but its main importance is in sustaining weight loss, and maintaining weight once the initial 5 or 10% loss has occurred. A study of policemen in the Boston area of the US (Paylou et al 1989) showed minimal difference in weight loss between diet alone and diet plus exercise, but only the exercise group sustained weight loss in the long term. Other studies confirm these findings, although measuring and assessing physical exercise is notoriously difficult and inaccurate, partly because self-reporting of exercise seems to be as wayward as self-reporting of food intake and partly because methods of correctly measuring activity during all phases, including vigorous and sedentary, is challenging.

So the best way to assess the medical and physiological benefits incurred by physical activity is *not* to become obsessed by the exact number of kilograms lost. Studies (Ballor & Poehlman 1994, Garrow & Summerbell 1995) show that the actual additional amount of weight lost by diet and physical activity, rather than diet alone, can be relatively minor, but that the medical benefits of physical activity are massive. This might be because regular exercise induces an increase in muscle bulk at the expense of fat, and therefore the fat-free mass increases: muscle weighs one-and-a-half times as much as fat and so actual body weight might be maintained or even increased when patients start performing unaccustomed exercise. However, muscle is a much healthier substance to fill our bodies with than fat, having fewer of the dangers and the advantage of increasing metabolic rate (compared with the usual reduction of BMR that occurs with weight loss), thus aiding concurrent dietary efforts to lose weight. A person who is becoming fitter by increasing his or her exercise levels is likely to show a decrease in waist circumference despite maintaining constant weight, and it can be valuable to demonstrate changes in body composition by, for instance, bioelectrical impedance analysis (BIA) as an illustration to the patient that all the hard work is worthwhile.

Physical activity has significant health benefits regardless of whether or not weight loss occurs. These are listed in *Box 6.2*.

Physical activity is therefore a vital component in the battle against overweight and obesity, but its benefit cannot simply be measured in pounds and ounces – it is much broader than this, resulting in independent improvement in comorbidities, as well as improved overall physical fitness.

6.21 How does exercise lead to weight loss?

For the purposes of weight loss, the best type of exercise is low to medium intensity, which uses the oxidation of free fatty acids as its energy supply. Exercise such as swimming, brisk walking, gardening or wheeling oneself in

---

BOX 6.2 Advantages of physical activity

- ■ Improved control of type 2 diabetes
- ■ Improved lipid profile, in particular an increase in high-density lipoprotein levels (Wood et al 1991)
- ■ Improved blood pressure (Krotkiewski et al 1979)
- ■ Improved insulin sensitivity (Helmrich et al 1991)
- ■ Improved self-esteem and reduction in symptoms of depression and anxiety (Morgan 1997)
- ■ Improved day-to-day functional capacity
- ■ Reduced risk of colorectal cancer because of altered metabolism of environmental carcinogens

---

a wheelchair to burn off fat, combined with a reduced-fat diet, is a good recipe for weight loss, and especially maintenance of weight loss. More vigorous exercise such as squash, sprinting or lifting heavy weights uses glycogen stores from the liver as its energy source in preference to fat, which, although highly beneficial for cardiovascular fitness, does not lead to weight loss as successfully.

The more prolonged the exercise, the more oxidation of fat occurs for use as an energy source and there is evidence that fat stores are oxidized after prolonged bouts of exercise to top-up reduced glycogen stores. These facts are leading to subtle changes in the recommendations for exercise for weight control; although 30 minutes per day has been shown to have benefits, more prolonged exercise has a greater benefit for the depletion of fat stores, suggesting that periods of exercise should be maintained for longer. The frequency of exercise is important; bouts of exercise only once or twice a week are beneficial, but only affect fat oxidation during that exercise and briefly afterwards, whereas exercise five or more times a week enables us to oxidize fats more efficiently on a more permanent basis.

Equally important is the effect of exercise on appetite, which is reduced immediately after exercise. However, after vigorous exercise there is a tendency for the appetite to increase after rest and rehydration and this, combined with a smug certainty that food is well-deserved, often results in eating. Food intake at this stage causes immediate replenishing of glycogen reserves and minimizes weight loss. After sustained low-intensity exercise, it appears that the effect on appetite is less and therefore the likelihood of immediate replacement of calories is less, and more easily resisted.

Appetite is also controlled by long-term fitness levels: 'fit' people who exercise regularly have a 'normal' appetite, whereas sedentary 'unfit' people have lost regulatory control over their appetite because they lack the normal stimuli and exercise pattern ingrained upon us during our hunting and gathering past. The exact reasons are not known; Blundell & King (1998) suggested that active people rely on hunger to tell them when to eat and thus control their food intake, whereas inactive individuals rely on satiety to tell them when they've had enough. It is thought that hunger is more efficient as a physiological mechanism, and therefore as a weight control as well.

6.22 What are the current recommendations for physical activity?

Current guidelines suggest that, health permitting, obese adults should endeavour to perform 30 minutes of increased exercise per day *in addition* to their normal daily routine. The 30 minutes can be cumulative – made up of 10- or 15-minute bursts – or carried out in one go: continuing for more than 30 minutes is beneficial if one is accustomed to increased levels of exercise. However, The WHO report *Diet, nutrition and prevention of chronic diseases*, published in April 2003, assessed all the latest up-to-date evidence and concluded that 45 to 60 minutes of exercise on most days are needed to prevent unhealthy weight gain and that between 60 and 90 minutes per day are required to prevent weight regain after substantial loss. It doesn't matter whether the extra time is made up at home, in the gym or in the shopping centre as long as it is additional activity, preferably enjoyable, and likely to be maintained permanently to avoid rebound weight gain.

Our daily ration of physical activity is split between normal day-to-day exertion – housework, daily work routine, washing the car, gardening and so on – and specifically scheduled physical exercise. Although many people might feel that they are fit because they can cope with their daily tasks without being tired or unduly short of breath, the truth is that their day-to-day tasks might be so physically mundane that they do not cause sufficient exertion to expose their lack of fitness.

Individuals with sedentary occupations should ensure that periods of sitting are broken at least every 30 minutes by some form of activity. For the purpose of weight loss in obese people, the most effective sort of exercise is aerobic, rather than vigorous or explosive exercise. This is partly because of the added cardiovascular risk of unaccustomed vigorous exercise and partly because the aim of exercise is to burn off fat stores (*see Q 6.21*). The optimum degree of exertion is said to be that of 'brisk exercise', which raises the pulse, causes sweating and quickened breathing, but the person can still talk. Although many people tend to increase their levels of activity at the weekends, by playing sport or spending active time with a young family, it is important to remember that many people who are active from Monday to Friday at work do the opposite, and will relax and do little physical activity at weekends. Advice on physical activity should stress that, beneficial as extra exertion at work may be, the increased levels should continue at weekends when there is often more time to donate to physical pursuits.

6.23 How is physical activity measured?

Levels of physical activity are measured by personal interview, to make estimates of total energy levels. However, it is recognized that people often over-report how much physical activity they do. Much more reliable are Computer Science Applications (CSA) accelerometers. These can record all movements undertaken and, when subsequently downloaded onto a computer, show detailed patterns of physical activity during the day.

Fox et al (BNF 1999) have shown some fascinating patterns of physical activity. Overall, girls appear to have lower levels of physical activity than boys at school, being less active at playtime. However, boys are much less active than girls after school and at weekends. Fox et al compared the physical activity levels of obese boys with those of normal-weight boys. The obese boys tended to be less active throughout the school day and even less active than their normal-weight peers over the weekend. Whether lower levels of activity have contributed to their obesity, or their obesity to their lower levels of activity is unclear. These data would suggest that the role of physical activity within the school curriculum is perhaps more important than has been previously appreciated.

Another crude method of measurement, which has with simple clinical applications, is to measure physical activity using a pedometer. A pedometer is a small, inexpensive piece of equipment, usually attached to the belt, which monitors the number of steps taken. As a rough guide, 2000 steps equates to one kilometre of walking. To achieve weight maintenance, it is recommended that 7000 steps are taken each day and in those who wish to lose weight, 10 000 steps are recommended. A pedometer can provide a useful measure for patients wishing to monitor their physical activity, and indeed for those who are trying to increase it.

6.24 Can you be fat and fit?

There are clear benefits of physical activity, quite apart from the levels of body fat. Physical activity has been shown to reduce the risk of coronary heart disease, stroke and hypertension, improve the blood lipid profile, improve the management of type 2 diabetes, reduce blood pressure, reduce the risk of osteoporosis, low back pain, and even reduce the risk of some cancers. Some studies have suggested that highly active individuals with several cardiovascular risk factors have similar levels of mortality as those without cardiovascular risk factors but who are inactive.

Obese individuals can decrease their overall risk by becoming more physically active, even in the absence of weight loss. It is far better to gain the benefits of weight loss at the same time but it does indeed appear to be possible for an individual to be 'fat and fit'.

6.25 Does increased physical activity assist weight loss?

Increased physical activity on its own is a poor inducer of weight loss. Exercise alone will produce on average weight loss of around 0.5 kg per month, much less than compared to dietary approaches alone. An individual who attempts to 'burn-off' body fat by regular, intense exercise might find that, despite their efforts, weight loss does not occur. One explanation for this is that although total body fat mass might decrease, the exercise encourages the development of increased lean muscle mass. Muscle weighs more than an equivalent amount of fat and so weight loss may not occur. In such individuals, it might be more encouraging to monitor waist circumference or total body fat mass as a better indicator of 'fat-loss'. Although exercise is undoubtedly to be encouraged, by far the best weight loss results are achieved when dietary adjustment and increased activity are combined. Studies show that not only are those who are more physically active more likely to lose weight, but they are also more likely to maintain their weight loss long term. It is quite rare for an individual to sustain long-term weight loss without maintaining increased physical activity levels (*see also Q 6.20*).

6.26 What is the effect of exercise on childhood obesity?

Life in the twenty-first century has affected our children just as much, if not more, than it has affected adults. The morning walk to school is a thing of the past as parents have become increasingly concerned about the threats of pollution, increasing traffic on the roads, joyriders and so-called 'Stranger Danger' paedophiles living round the corner. Physical activity at school has plummeted as playing fields have been sold off to boost school funds, competitive sports have been labelled as socially and politically unacceptable and local education authorities have bowed to an increasingly litigious society by not putting children at the slightest risk of injury.

In 1990, Armstrong et al demonstrated that almost 50% of girls and 38% of boys did not achieve one 10-minute period of exercise equivalent to brisk walking, in three school days, although the Health and Lifestyle Survey 1991 (Health Education Authority 1991) was more optimistic, revealing that 9 to 15-year-olds are, on average, involved in 4.7 hours of exercise per week.

Equally alarming are the statistics showing what goes on outside schools; in 1971 half of our children were allowed to travel to school by bus on their own; in 1990 the number was one in seven. Between 1986 and 1996 the number of car journeys to school doubled (National Audit Office 2002). The home is safer and more comfortable than ever; children can feed and entertain themselves fully without setting foot outside the front door; on average they watch almost 3 hours of TV per day and many have TVs in their bedroom, so don't even have to go to the trouble of getting out of bed. To make matters worse, many children snack on crisps and biscuits while viewing, adding hundreds of extra calories to the equation, a fact that has escaped neither the TV networks nor the food industry, which advertises its wares at maximum intensity during children's TV programmes. If TV becomes a bore then there are ever more computer games to play, with ever increasing complexity, requiring more and more practice to reach the final goal. Gortmaker et al (1996) calculated that the risk of overweight is 4.6 times higher in children who watch more than 5 hours of TV per day (*Fig. 6.3*). Epstein et al (1995) revealed that reducing sedentary occupations such as TV watching is more beneficial as a means of weight management than attempting to introduce vigorous activity sessions.

6.27 What is being done to change the situation?

After consulting across the range of government departments and healthcare providers in the UK, the National Audit Office (NAO) produced a report full of good ideas to 'overcome specific barriers to physical activity, such as those imposed by poverty, cultural beliefs or fears about personal safety' (NAO 2002 p 20). However, unless specific steps are taken to bring

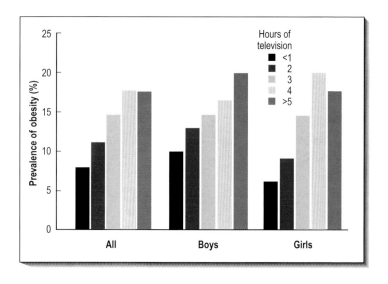

▲
Fig. 6.3 Time spent viewing television is related to the degree of overweight in children (from Crespo et al 2001).

these ideas out of the conference room, they are of little value. *Box 6.3* highlights the recommendations of the NAO report.

A health promotion study in Glasgow included in the NAO report involved placing a sign at the bottom of the escalators on the underground saying 'Stay healthy, save time, use the stairs'; use of the stairs increased from 8% to 16% and stayed at the higher level even after the signs were removed.

6.28 Are 'fat camps' good or bad?

The expression 'fat camps' refers to residential activity programmes, usually for obese children and adolescents, which involve increased levels of activity with the aim of weight loss. Critics argue that because the camps are only brief excursions away from the child's usual obesogenic environment, any reduction in body weight is only short term and will reverse when the person returns to normal day-to-day life. They also comment that attendees are self-selecting and are therefore the minority of children who have both the motivation and the money to take part.

Paul Gately set up such a camp in Leeds. He believes that residential courses are successful and have a place in modern management of obesity. He argues that weight-loss diets are potentially unsafe in children and so increased activity is essential, and that management strategies combining dietary education, behavioural modification, a reduction in sedentary pursuits and an increase in physical activity are likely to succeed. The emphasis in camps such as the Leeds one is on enjoyment of activity, so there is a good chance it will continue when the child returns home. There are three elements:

BOX 6.3 Recommendations of the National Audit Office report on overcoming the barriers to physical activity

- At least 2 hours physical activity a week for all school pupils
- A joint advisory group to monitor the success of initiatives to increase physical activity in schools
- Exercise on prescription to increase from the 200 referral-based schemes operating in 1998
- A safer and more integrated network of appropriate routes, footpaths and cycle lanes
- Encouraging people to reconsider their car and adopt healthier modes of transport such as cycling and walking
- Broadening the range of activities schools can offer to encourage young people to participate in different forms of physical recreation

- fun-type exercise and physical activities
- skill development in the physical activities
- exposure of children to a wide range of physical activities with a strong element of choice.

Studies performed at the camp reveal favourable changes in body mass, adiposity and other risk factors (Gately & Cooke 2003), enabling optimistic predictions for the future of fat camps.

6.29 What is meant by 'microactivity'?

'Microactivity' is a term that has been coined to describe the minor, apparently trivial movements and tasks that occur to a greater or lesser extent throughout our daily lives. An opposite term – 'macroactivity' – describes the tasks we perform; microactivity is the sum of the small detailed movements comprising those tasks.

A task can be performed using the minimum possible energy output or it can be embellished, depending on the intensity of the underlying microactivity. It is estimated that standing or sitting immobile, for instance during a telephone call, burns off approximately one calorie per minute, whereas talking on the phone while pottering around the living room increases the number of calories burnt by two- or three-fold. It has also been estimated that to sustain weight loss requires a calorie deficit of 150 kcal per day on average, compared to a person's previous intake. Therefore walking while on the phone enables a person to sustain weight loss.

Other examples of microactivity range from 'fidgeting' movements of the legs, hand rubbing and head scratching, to walking up and down the train platform, going upstairs on the bus and even hand gesticulations during speech. Other examples are dwindling with the advent of technology: pushing doors open uses more energy than using an automatic door, TV remote controls allow us to sit undisturbed, central locking in cars is far less effort than manual. Nevertheless, activity can be fitted into daily life much more. Those people who never seem to sit still for a minute and who fidget, wave their arms and twiddle their thumbs are maximizing their microactivity levels and burning off calories more rapidly than those who stay still.

6.30 What can be done to improve activity levels?

It is often said that 'you can lead a horse to water but you can't make it drink'. Equally, should the horse want water, it can only drink if water is provided within a reasonable distance. In other words, simply informing people about the need for more physical activity will not produce any positive results unless there is adequate provision for their needs. Encouraging people to cycle to work is unlikely to make much difference unless there are designated cycle lanes to make their journey safe and more enjoyable. Encouraging parents to allow their children to walk to school is unlikely to have much of an impact unless we can simultaneously make the roads safer from the threat of cars and the fear of abduction felt by so many parents. People are unlikely to leave their cars at home if the provision of public transport is inadequate or if that public transport is inconvenient, expensive and unreliable.

Much could be done within schools to increase the amount of time spent in PE lessons and to increase the level of enjoyment experienced by children during that physical activity. Sport and physical activity need to be made more attractive to adolescents, particularly girls, and the increased activity needs to be carried into adulthood. Parents should be more aware of the harmful effects of prolonged TV watching or computer game play and be encouraged to limit the amount of time their children spend on these activities. Individuals attempting to lose weight need more support and guidance on physical activity, what levels are safe and appropriate, and what levels are appropriate for their individual weight-loss programmes.

6.31 How should the chronically ill increase their activity levels?

It is important to gear the recommendations on activity to the individual, rather than setting unrealistic goals. An increase in activity levels is important, however little:

- For obese chronic bronchitics, a brief potter in the garden every hour might represent a significant increase in activity.
- Asthmatic patients might need to be advised to take their salbutamol inhaler prior to exercising.
- For arteriopaths, a walk up and down stairs might be appropriate
- For anyone with severe physical limitations, advice such as 'stand up when talking on the phone' might be enough.

The US Surgeon General's report (see http://www.surgeongeneral.gov/topics/obesity) recommends wheeling oneself in a wheelchair for 40 minutes as being a reasonable level of activity for health benefits, whereas a patient with lower-limb orthopaedic problems may be advised to perform low-impact activities.

6.32 Is inactivity a health risk?

One of the main causes of obesity is physical inactivity but there is convincing evidence that physical inactivity should be considered in its own right as an independent risk factor for disease. Inactivity is obviously more prevalent in obese people but the two are not mutually exclusive and can be considered separately. The evidence for this is based on the fact that even when there is no reduction in weight, parameters such as blood pressure, lipid levels and insulin sensitivity can still be improved by reducing sedentary behaviour. Moreover, non-obese people derive significant health benefits from decreasing periods of inactivity, indicating that activity is essential, obese or not.

In fact, the risk carried by inactivity alone is massive. Powell et al (1987) judged that inactivity alone causes a two-fold risk for all-cause mortality, and follows hard on the heels of smoking and hypertension in terms of damage done. It has been suggested, and widely accepted, that inactivity can be considered as the fourth primary risk factor for stroke and coronary heart disease.

The concept that 'fit and fat' is better than 'lean and unfit' is controversial, unprovable and probably mainly peddled by 'fit, fat' individuals, but it is nevertheless sensible that, fat or lean, it is better to be fit. However, Lee et al 1998 have shown that active obese people have a much reduced risk for mortality and morbidity than their obese and inactive peers.

In practice, it not uncommon to see obese people who have gone to considerable effort to lose weight by physical activity and who are verging on inconsolable when the needle on the scales hasn't shifted for weeks. It should be stressed to them that because of their increased activity, their fitness *will* have improved, which is one key outcome of treatment. If such a person is told that having increased activity levels does nearly as much for them as giving up smoking, they are likely to go away a little less despondent.

BEHAVIOURAL THERAPY

6.33 What is behavioural therapy?

If, during a weight-loss programme, one arrives home from a stressful day at work and heads immediately for the cupboard for two comforting chocolate biscuits, basic dietary and nutritional advice might be 'don't eat those chocolate biscuits'; behavioural therapy would suggest ways *how* not to eat the chocolate biscuits, in other words how to avoid them. The answer could be very simple: 'don't buy any chocolate biscuits' or more complex: 'avoid the stressful situation that triggered the desire for the chocolate biscuit', which might mean changing jobs or walking home instead of getting a crowded bus. Other suggestions might include not putting the biscuits where they are easy to reach and have readily accessible healthy snacks, such as fruit, to hand. Alternatively, there might be other ways to unwind: having a bath or swearing at the cat.

'Behavioural therapy' is the collective name for the various methods and strategies used to bring about changes in lifestyle. Behavioural techniques should always be combined with traditional dietary and activity advice to maximize the benefits and improve compliance with lifestyle change. More structured programmes of cognitive behavioural therapy (CBT) lasting for 4 or 5 months have been developed.

6.34 How successful is behavioural therapy?

In short-term studies, CBT has been shown to induce weight loss of 10% or more, but with less successful long-term results. Behavioural therapy as part of a programme of long-term support coupled with regular physical activity and dietary advice has been shown to be a lot more successful. Similarly, CBT combined with VLCD has produced significant weight loss (Wadden 1993).

6.35 What is meant by 'stages of change'?

In the context of weight management, 'stages of change' refers to the state of mind of the obese person and is a reflection of how motivated he or she is to undergo management for the condition. The six stages (*Fig. 6.4*) are:

1. Precontemplation: absolutely no chance of behavioural change.
2. Contemplation: awareness that there is a health problem and that something really should be done about it one day.
3. Preparation: awareness is acute and something is going to be done in the next month.

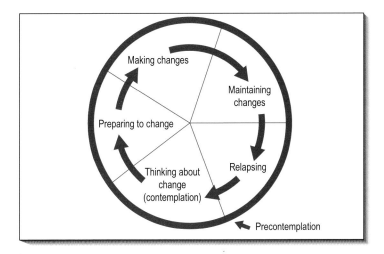

Fig. 6.4 The process of change (from Prochaska & DiClemente 1986, with permission).

4. Active change: behaviour is actively being modified to overcome the problem.
5. Maintenance: active change has been successful and consolidation and maintenance are taking place.
6. Relapse: back to stage one.

Before initiating treatment, it is important to recognize which stage the individual is at and to act accordingly. Management is unlikely to succeed if the wrong approach is made at the wrong time.

6.36 What does the language of behavioural therapy mean?

Different aspects of behavioural therapy have been analysed in minute detail and a whole language of terms and descriptions has been invented, but many of the concepts are simple and effective. Brownell (1997) described a range of skills and strategies, including self-monitoring, stimulus control, relapse management, social support and challenging negative thinking. Many of these techniques are summarized in *Table 6.2*.

Self-monitoring is a fundamental pillar of CBT. In its most basic form this constitutes a food and activity diary of what is eaten, where and in what circumstances, and what emotional feelings or triggers might have been involved. The diary should also contain a note of what levels of activity were performed. A food diary should clarify eating patterns and behaviours, especially the events that trigger eating, with a view to changing those patterns once they have been identified, for instance by planning ahead. Once the pattern of eating has been established by recording it in the food diary, the diary can be used as part of the treatment plan, by recording progress towards dietary goals. Long-term weight management has been shown to improve when food records are used (Baker & Kirschenbaum 1993).

'Stimulus control' refers to the different stimuli we have for eating, only one of which is feeling physically hungry. Eating chocolate biscuits on arriving home from work is more likely to be because of stress than hunger; the stimulus control therefore is remove the biscuit, or remove the stress. Other stimuli for eating are described as 'external cues'; these include:

■ time: eating because its lunchtime
■ presence of food: eating food because it is there or finishing a plateful because it is rude or wasteful not to
■ social cues: eating cheese and biscuits with a glass of port because everyone else is.

Stimulus control might involve avoiding external cues, for instance choosing a route home to avoid passing the Indian takeaway. Controlling eating at the last stage of the chain, for example when one is already looking

TABLE 6.2A Techniques of behaviour modification for weight management (from Brownell 1997).

Stimulus control	Self-monitoring	Eating behaviour	Rewards
Shopping: ■ Shop for food only on a full stomach ■ Shop from a list ■ Only buy appropriate foods ■ Avoid ready-to-eat foods ■ Only carry the amount of cash needed for foods on the shopping list *Plans:* ■ Plan to limit food intake ■ Pre-plan meals and snacks ■ Substitute exercise for snacking ■ Eat meals and snacks at scheduled times ■ Don't accept food offered by others *Activities:* ■ Use graphs, cartoons, pictures and so on to remind yourself to eat properly ■ Make nutritionally acceptable foods as attractive as possible in preparation and presentation ■ Remove inappropriate foods from the house ■ Store problem foods out of sight ■ Keep healthier foods visible ■ Eat all food in the same place ■ Remove food from inappropriate storage areas in the house	*Keep a dietary diary that includes:* ■ Time and place of eating ■ Type and amount of food ■ Who else (if anyone) is present ■ How you felt before eating ■ Activities that you are doing at the same time ■ Calories and/or fat contents of foods ■ Patterns in your eating	*Slow rate of eating:* ■ Take one small bite at a time ■ Chew food thoroughly before swallowing ■ Put fork down between mouthfuls ■ Pause in the middle of the meal and assess hunger *Do nothing else while eating:* ■ Concentrate on act of eating ■ Concentrate on enjoying food ■ Eat all food in one place ■ Follow eating plan	■ Solicit help from family and friends ■ Ask family and friends to provide this help in the form of praise and material rewards ■ Clearly define behaviours to be rewarded ■ Utilize self-monitoring records as basis for rewards ■ Plan specific rewards for specific behaviours ■ Gradually make rewards more difficult to achieve

TABLE 6.2A Techniques of behaviour modification for weight management (from Brownoll 1997).—cont'd

Stimulus control	Self-monitoring	Eating behaviour	Rewards
Serving food: ■ Keep serving dishes off the table ■ Use smaller dishes and utensils ■ Avoid being the food server ■ Serve and eat one portion at a time ■ Leave the table immediately after eating ■ Save leftovers for another meal instead of finishing what is on your plate *Holidays and parties:* ■ Prepare in advance what you will do ■ Drink fewer alcoholic beverages ■ Plan eating habits before parties ■ Eat a low-calorie snack before parties ■ Practise polite ways of declining food ■ Don't get discouraged by an occasional setback			

TABLE 6.2B Techniques of behaviour modification for weight management (from Brownoll 1997).

Nutrition education	Physical activity	Cognitive restructuring	Relapse management
■ Use self-monitoring diary to identify problem areas ■ Make small changes that can be continued ■ Eat a well-balanced diet ■ Learn nutritional values of food ■ Decrease fat intake, increase complex carbohydrate intake	*Lifestyle activity:* ■ Increase lifestyle activity ■ Increase use of stairs ■ Walk where you would normally use a bus/car ■ Keep a record of frequency, intensity and duration of time spent walking each day *Exercise:* ■ Start a mild exercise programme ■ Keep a record of daily exercise ■ Increase the amount of exercise very gradually	■ Develop realistic expectations of weight loss ■ Set reasonable, realistic weight-loss and behaviour-change goals ■ Focus on progress, not shortcomings ■ Avoid imperatives such as 'always' or 'never' ■ Keep a record of thoughts about self and weight ■ Challenge and counter self-defeating thoughts with positive thoughts	■ View lapses as opportunities to learn more about behaviour change ■ Identify triggers for lapsing ■ Plan in advance how to prevent lapses ■ Generate a list of coping strategies in high-risk situations ■ Distinguish hunger from cravings ■ Make a list of activities to do which make it impossible to give in to cravings ■ Confront or ignore cravings ■ Outlast urges to eat

at the menu in the curry-house window, is notoriously difficult, whereas taking action earlier in the chain, when the Indian meal is less tangible, is easier. The answer: take a different route home.

In the 1980s, Margaret Thatcher, the former British Prime Minister got into hot water when she suggested that people on low incomes should avoid shopping when they were hungry. She might have chosen the wrong time and place to mention it but, rightly or wrongly, she was teaching stimulus control. Other stimuli such as stress or emotional eating could be described as 'internal cues'.

'Learned self-control' becomes important when the only route home passes the Indian takeaway, or perhaps a Chinese takeaway is opened along the other route home, making external temptation unavoidable. Learned self-control occurs with prolonged repetition of the external stimulus, without giving in and eating. After enough journeys home without buying a takeaway, the conditioned response (i.e. buying a takeaway because you are passing the restaurant) will diminish.

'Stress management' is self-explanatory: comfort foods are widely recognized as a substrate for overeating. However, there is conflicting evidence for 'hyperphagia' in the presence of a stressful environment and stress will often cause loss of appetite.

6.37 When did behavioural therapy for obesity originate?

Behavioural therapy for obesity originated in the 1950s and 1960s, at the same time that Dr Albert Stunkard was beginning to realize that binge eaters and night eaters would not respond to simply being told to 'go on a diet' but needed profound counselling and psychological help. The theory put forward at the time was that obesity was caused by an 'obese eating style'. Therapy would ensure a return to normal body weight by eliminating abnormal eating behaviour, and normal weight would be sustained permanently (Ferster et al 1962). Although this has clearly not occurred, behavioural techniques have improved and the advent of CBT in the 1970s, which identified and changed negative thoughts, has played an important role in the long-term management of obesity.

It is now possible to undergo behavioural therapy via the internet (Tate et al 2001). It has been demonstrated that websites that include behavioural techniques induce greater weight loss than information sites alone.

6.38 How does alcohol intake affect weight?

Heavy alcohol intake is closely linked with obesity, and people who start drinking heavily will tend to gain weight rapidly. Although the common assumption is that beer drinkers will end up with increased abdominal girth and 'beer bellies', the phenomenon appears to be the same whatever the form of alcohol consumed (Wannamethee & Shaper 2003).

6.39 Is there a link between obesity and dental health?

Obese young adults have twice the risk of gum disease than middle- and older-aged adults according to studies done in the American and Japanese populations, and the prevalence of periodontal disease is 76% higher among young obese individuals than in young normal-weight ones. How much the dental disease is due to the eating of high-calorie foods and sugary foods, and how much to other factors is unclear (Al-Zarahni et al 2003).

PATIENT QUESTIONS

6.40   Can obesity be linked with eating disorders?

Yes: some patterns of overeating have the characteristics of an eating disorder. Many people eat for reasons other than hunger – stress, excitement, loneliness and 'comfort eating'. Sometimes this can be taken to extremes. People with binge eating disorder suffer from prolonged episodes during which they have no control over what they eat and will consume vast quantities before stopping. Night eating syndrome is characterized by eating frequently in the evening and during the night but by loss of appetite for breakfast and lunch. People with these conditions should be offered therapy for their eating disorder in addition to straightforward weight-loss advice if they are to succeed in losing weight.

6.41   Which is the best diet?

There is no such thing as 'the best diet', as different methods suit different individuals; what works for you might not work for your next door neighbour. Although the various diets each have their own rules and ideas, which make them unique, a diet will really only work if it induces you to eat fewer calories than before. There is no secret formula or magic food combination to improve your metabolism or make the body work better, the answer is that a successful diet is one that enables you to have a smaller intake of energy. So, rather than choosing a commercial diet, and trying to stick to it for as long as possible, it is better to learn about food and nutrition to be able to choose better foods and to use healthy cooking methods to adapt your diet in a manner that you can stick to for the rest of your life. It is worthwhile looking at the labels on food packaging and being aware which foods are genuinely low in fat, sugar, salt and additives, and avoiding unhealthy foods. Many slimming organizations and clubs, and internet weight-loss sites, include education and awareness of food and nutrition as a central part of their work.

6.42   How much exercise should I take?

All activity is good. A person should take as much exercise during the day-to-day routine as possible by, for instance, walking or cycling instead of catching a bus, walking up the escalator or stairs instead of taking a lift, walking a bit further to buy lunch and avoiding long periods seated at a desk or computer. It is also important to get extra exercise outside the daily routine, by going for a walk or a swim, or playing sports, although vigorous exercise should be introduced gradually. It is thought that, to keep fit, 30 minutes of exercise per day is reasonable but that to lose weight, or prevent weight being regained, up to 90 minutes is necessary.

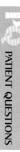

Management: pharmacotherapy

7

7.1   Do drugs have a role in obesity management?

The vast majority of patients embarking on a weight-loss programme will not require treatment with weight-loss medication. The key to long-term successful weight loss must be significant and sustained lifestyle change. However, it is evident from clinical experience and extensive research that, even with the best professional support, a significant proportion of patients cannot achieve medically beneficial weight loss (5–10% body weight loss). The use of medication as an aid to weight loss can significantly increase the number of patients achieving medically beneficial weight loss.

7.2   What role do drugs have in weight maintenance?

The ideal outcome of any weight-loss programme must be long-term weight maintenance. It is well recognized that many patients struggle to maintain weight loss after a period of time. The level of clinical support offered can dramatically alter the long-term outcome and the more frequently contacts with health professionals occur, the more likely the patient is to succeed at weight maintenance after the initial phase of weight loss. A cessation or even a reduction in clinical contacts can leave many patients without the resolve to continue their newly modified dietary and exercise habits.

After the initial weight loss phase of 3–6 months the majority of patients experience a phase of weight maintenance, or even some weight gain. This 'plateau' effect requires as much clinical support as the initial period of weight loss if a reversal is to be prevented. Despite this, many patients will struggle. There has been extensive research into the use of medication in prolonging the phase of weight loss and increasing the likelihood of successful weight maintenance. Studies available to date show significant prolongation of weight maintenance for up to 4 years, when using medication.

7.3   When should drugs be used?

Medication can be considered for use as an adjunctive treatment to supported lifestyle changes in the following circumstances:
- After 3–6 months of compliance with dietary, behavioural and activity advice.
- If a patient has failed to achieve 10% loss of body weight.
- To enhance further reduction in symptomatology, such as breathlessness or weight-bearing joint pain.
- To achieve further improvements in markers of comorbidity, such as hyperlipidaemia or raised blood pressure.

> ■ To improve exercise tolerance and promote increased physical activity.
> ■ To improve diabetic control, lower fasting blood glucose and other diabetes indices.
> ■ For psychological reasons: for some patients, the support provided by medication can act as a powerful motivating factor, increasing their confidence to be more physically active and enhancing their desire and ability to exercise dietary restraint.

7.4   When are drugs inappropriate?

■ When the patient profile lies outside licensing guidelines.

■ When weight loss achieved through lifestyle change is satisfactory.

■ If a patient has a history of previous adverse reactions to the chosen medication.

■ Where there are contraindications to use of the chosen medication.

■ For non-medical motivating factors: e.g. for short-term weight loss prior to a holiday or a wedding.

■ When a patient fails to exhibit serious attempts at lifestyle modification.

■ With a recurrent history of cyclical (yo-yo) dieting.

■ When a patient has unrealistic expectations of excessive weight loss.

■ With a history of eating disorders such as anorexia nervosa or bulimia.

Underlying psychological or psychiatric disorders should be addressed prior to any contemplation of the use of medication, but their use might be appropriate after further, sometimes specialist, assessment.

7.5   What drugs are currently available?

> Several agents are currently available and used by medical practitioners to aid weight loss. There are, however, only two agents currently recommended and licensed for use in Europe for the long-term treatment of obesity:
> ■ orlistat (Xenical®)
> ■ sibutramine (Europe: Reductil®, US: Meridia®).

Orlistat first became available in the Europe in 1999. It is classified as an intestinal lipase inhibitor and prevents absorption of fats from the small intestine. Sibutramine has been available in some parts of Europe and the US since 1999, and in the UK since 2001. It acts centrally and is classified as a serotonin (5HT) reuptake inhibitor.

ORLISTAT

7.6   How does orlistat work?

Orlistat was developed to reduce the amount of dietary fat absorbed from the small intestine and so decrease an individual's total calorific intake. Acting locally to block the action of pancreatic and gastric lipase enzyme, it reduces absorption of fat – in particular triglycerides – by up to one-third. The unabsorbed dietary fat is excreted through the intestine.

The average fat content of a Western diet can be as high as 45% and contributes greatly to overall calorific intake. Reducing fat intake by dietary means can produce significant benefits. However, further reductions in dietary fat absorption can be achieved by the addition of orlistat, thereby achieving further net decreases in energy intake and contributing to a negative energy equation that can result in net weight loss. It is absolutely essential that the patient has been instructed in, and has adapted to, a low-fat diet before treatment is commenced.

7.7   How is orlistat taken?

Orlistat is prescribed as 120-mg capsules, one of which is to be taken three times a day during (or up to one hour after) meals. Patients must have been instructed in, and demonstrated that they can follow, a low-fat dietary regime. Failure to adhere to a low-fat diet can result in unpleasant side-effects and will lead to poor compliance and early cessation of treatment. If a meal is missed, the medication should be omitted. Some patients will choose to omit individual doses when eating out or when knowingly eating a high-fat meal. Patients taking vitamin supplements should ensure they do not take them within 2 hours of taking orlistat.

7.8   What are the potential side-effects of orlistat?

Because of its local mode of action, orlistat has no common systemic side-effects. If the patient fails to adhere to a low-fat diet (less than 30% calories taken in as fat) the inhibited intestinal absorption can lead to oily spotting, flatus, faecal urgency and anal leakage. Patients can be helped to view these effects positively, as 'treatment effects' and learn to adapt their dietary intake accordingly.

Occasionally, malabsorption of the fat-soluble vitamins A, D, E and K might occur, although this is not a practical risk in normal clinical practice or when a patient is limited to a prescription duration of 12 months. Some clinicians choose to prescribe vitamin supplements in those taking orlistat for more than 1 year.

7.9 Are there any contraindications to orlistat?

Orlistat is contraindicated in patients with cholestasis or malabsorptive syndromes. It should also not be used in patients who are unable to tolerate or maintain a low-fat diet (*see Q 7.8*).

7.10 Are any special precautions advised for orlistat?

 Treatment with orlistat can reduce vitamin K absorption so special attention is warranted in anticoagulated patients. Patients on warfarin therapy should have their international normalized ratio (INR) checked regularly.

Orlistat might also reduce the absorption of cyclosporin and it is therefore advisable to monitor blood levels. Despite initial concerns, there is no data to support the association of orlistat with breast cancer.

SIBUTRAMINE

7.11 How does sibutramine work?

Sibutramine was developed in the UK as a centrally acting, serotonin and noradrenaline reuptake inhibitor. Weight loss is facilitated by two actions:

■ Sibutramine's central action on neurotransmitters causes an enhancement of satiety (fullness) after eating, which results in a 20% reduction in overall calorific intake. It is not an appetite suppressant, loss of appetite being a listed side-effect occurring in less than 10% of patients prescribed sibutramine. Prolonged satiety does, however reduce the need for snacking between meals.

■ A second action is by sympathetically mediated thermogenesis, which prevents the reduction in basal metabolic rate (BMR) normally seen in individuals on restrictive diets and thereby effectively increases resting energy consumption and promotes weight loss. By virtue of its mode of action, it can cause some sympathetic stimulation and lead to unwanted cardiovascular changes.

7.12 How is sibutramine taken?

 Sibutramine is taken as a 10-mg capsule, once daily, usually in the morning. The dose can be increased to 15 mg daily after 1 month if there is insufficient weight loss (<2 kg), i.e. the patient is a 'poor responder'.

7.13 What are the potential side-effects of sibutramine?

The potential side-effects of sibutramine are easily understood from its mode of action (*see Q 7.11*). The most common side-effects, affecting about 10% of patients, are headache, dizziness, sweating, palpitations, constipation and dry mouth. There is an average rise in diastolic blood pressure of 2.3 mmHg, the average pulse rate rising by 3 beats per minute. A significant rise in pulse rate and blood pressure can be seen in some patients, usually in the first 3 months, requiring cessation of treatment. It is therefore necessary that patients are monitored closely for cardiovascular changes, particularly in the first 3 months of treatment.

7.14 Are there any contraindications to sibutramine?

Sibutramine should not be used in patients with a proven history of coronary heart disease, cardiac arrhythmias or uncontrolled hypertension. It should also be avoided in patients who have a history of stroke, heart failure, eating disorders or psychiatric illness and in those currently treated with antipsychotics or antidepressants.

7.15 Are any special precautions advised for sibutramine?

In early 2002, some concern was raised over the safety of sibutramine after the unexplained deaths of two patients in Italy. However, the European Committee for Proprietary Medicinal Products (CPMP) investigated sibutramine and concluded that it exhibits a positive favourable risk profile for the management of obesity.

Sibutramine can be used safely in well-controlled hypertensives (BP not greater than 145/90 mmHg) and in all patients blood pressure and pulse should be monitored every 2 weeks for the first 3 months of treatment, every 4 weeks for the following 3 months, and every 3 months thereafter. Treatment should be stopped if blood pressure rises by 10 mmHg on two consecutive readings or if the pulse rate rises by 10 beats per minute.

Data published by Abbott Laboratories Ltd suggest that blood pressure rises sufficiently to cause cessation of treatment in 10% of cases. Postmarketing surveillance studies from Austria have found that only 2% were sufficiently affected to require cessation of treatment on these grounds.

7.16 What is the difference between orlistat and sibutramine?

Table 7.1 provides a comparison of orlistat and sibutramine.

TABLE 7.1 Comparison of orlistat and sibutramine

	Orlistat	Sibutramine
Eligibility for treatment		
BMI >30	+	+
BMI ≥27 plus one comorbidity		+
BMI ≥28 plus one comorbidity	+	
Pretreatment requirements		
	Patient is required to display weight loss of at least 2.5 kg through lifestyle change in a preceding month. Low-fat diet essential (<30%)	Patient has been unable to display weight loss of at least 5% through lifestyle change within previous 3 months
Continuation of therapy		
1-month criteria		2-kg weight loss
3-month criteria	5% weight loss	5% weight loss
6-month criteria	10% weight loss	

Note: 'Comorbidity' includes diabetes, hyperlipidaemia, hypertension (sibutramine) and CHD (orlistat).

OTHER WEIGHT-LOSS DRUGS

7.17 What other prescribed agents can help effect weight loss?

Metformin has been shown to have advantageous effects in some diabetics trying to reduce their weight. Its effect on insulin resistance has been utilized in obese non-diabetic subjects to aid weight loss, and in particular in women who are overweight because of polycystic ovary syndrome (PCOS). Some practitioners have experimented by using it in combination with orlistat or sibutramine. It does not have any specific licensing arrangements for the treatment of obesity and currently does not have a clearly defined role.

7.18 What other types of drug have been used to help weight loss?

Clinicians have tried for decades to help patients lose weight with the aid of medication. *Box 7.1* lists those drugs that should not be used for weight loss.

Prior to the introduction of orlistat and sibutramine, the drugs available to aid weight loss were bulk-forming agents, such as methyl-cellulose, and centrally acting anorectics, such as phentermine.

Bulk-forming agents are rarely used now, quite simply because they don't work. Initial hopes that they could help patients decrease their dietary

> **BOX 7.1 Drugs that should not be used in a weight-loss programme**
>
> ■ Diuretics, amphetamine, dexamphetamine and thyroxine are not treatments for obesity and should never be used as such
> ■ Thyroxine should never be used in the management of obese patients in the absence of biochemically proven hypothyroidism
> ■ SSRI antidepressant drugs can be used to treat depression in obese patients but should not be considered as weight-loss drugs

intake by creating a feeling of fullness have not been realized in clinical studies or in clinical experience.

Centrally acting antiobesity drugs generally act in the brain to increase the release of serotonin and noradrenaline, resulting in decreased appetite. They act either on the serotonin pathways or on the catecholaminergic pathways. The most commonly used anorectic agent of recent years has been phentermine.

The centrally acting anorectics are virtually unused within the NHS, their last few remaining outlets being predominantly through private slimming clinics. The anorectic agents fenfluoramine and dexfenfluoramine fell out of use in 1997 after being withdrawn by the manufacturers. Phentermine and amfepramone have been serially licensed, withdrawn, reinstated, withdrawn and reinstated yet again. Currently, the manufacturers of phentermine and amfepramone are still engaged in legal disputes with the European regulatory authority, the CPMP, and their ultimate status is currently undecided. These drugs are discussed in detail below.

7.19 What prescribed drugs can promote weight gain?

Drugs that can promote weight gain are listed in *Box 7.2*.

7.20 What is phentermine?

Phentermine is a centrally acting, catecholaminergic drug that produces a decrease in appetite that can help patients decrease their food intake. After being swallowed it produces peak plasma concentrations within 8 hours and its therapeutic effect might last for 20 hours.

Phentermine has mild to moderate stimulant properties and its side-effects are related to this: headache, dry mouth, constipation, fast pulse, sweating and restlessness. The dosage is usually 15 to 30 mg, taken each morning. Withdrawal effects can lead to depression and lethargy.

There is no published literature to suggest that phentermine results in drug dependence, particularly if used for no more than the licensed 3-month period. However, there is little evidence to support the use of

---

BOX 7.2 Drugs that can promote weight gain

- Antipsychotics, especially olanzepine (Zyprexa®)
- Antidepressants: tricyclics, SSRIs, MAOIs, mirtazepine (Zispin®) and lithium
- Corticosteroids: promote weight gain by two mechanisms. (i) Fat redistribution causing truncal obesity, buffalo hump and moon face; and (ii) fluid retention via mineralocorticoid effects
- Oral contraceptive and progesterogenic compounds
- Beta-blockers: not only do these agents cause weight gain, they might also restrict physical activity due to fatigue
- Oral hypoglycaemics: numerous agents have been shown to increase weight, including the glitazones. Sulphonylureas (except glimepiride) have been shown to increase weight by an average of 2–4 kg but by as much as 10 kg in some cases
- Insulin
- Anticonvulsants: weight gain has been documented with some agents (phenytoin, sodium valproate). However, topiramate (Topamax) is weight neutral or may cause weight loss
- Antihistamines: many antihistamines might cause weight gain, although this is more pronounced in older agents
- Pizotifen: a prophylactic migraine treatment, pizotifen increases the appetite and leads to weight gain

---

phentermine beyond 3 months as there are insufficient recent data to support its efficacy and safety beyond a 3-month period. It is therefore difficult to justify routine use of phentermine as it is commonly considered that 3 months drug treatment is insufficient to produce meaningful and sustained weight loss with supported lifestyle change.

7.21 Why were the licences of anorectic agents withdrawn?

Serious concerns about the long-term effects of fenfluoramine and dexfenfluoramine had been raised as early as 1997. They were implicated in the development of heart valve defects, particularly when used in combination (a fenfluoramine–phentermine combination known in the US as fen-phen had been extremely popular). Defects of mitral and aortic valves were found, some symptomatic, others only on echocardiogram, with prevalence rates as high as 13% in one study. Accordingly, in 1997, fenfluoramine and dexfenfluoramine were voluntarily withdrawn by the manufacturers. There were also well-documented cases of primary pulmonary hypertension (PPH) associated with fenfluoramine, dexfenfluoramine and phentermine when used in isolation. These were associated with prolonged use (greater than 3 months) and cumulative dosing. Although often reversible, some cases were fatal.

On 9 April 2000, the European Committee for Proprietary Medicines (CPMP) published a review of the risks and benefits of the anorectic agents phentermine and amfepramone. It was widely publicized in the medical and national press that the CPMP had withdrawn the license for both agents. Clinicians were advised to cease initiating treatment with the drugs and to withdraw existing treated patients over a period of several weeks to minimize the possible effects of drug withdrawal. The manufacturers requested pharmacies and stock-holders to return their supplies to their wholesalers. However, by the middle of April 2000 the manufacturers of both drugs appealed to the European Courts and challenged the decision of the CPMP on the withdrawal of their license. The appeal was successful and by 7 August 2000, both phentermine and amfepramone had their licenses reinstated and once more became widely available. During the time the drugs were unlicensed, they remained available on a named-patient basis and continued to be used widely within the private slimming clinic industry. Their use within the NHS, already limited, ceased almost completely.

7.22 What is the current legal status of the anorectic agents?

Since August 2000 there has been a great deal of confusion about the legal status of phentermine and amfepramone. In May 2001 the manufacturers' appeal was overturned in the European courts and the suspension of the original decision was set aside. The Medicines Control Agency (MCA) in the UK advised a second withdrawal of the drugs. It was noted that this second withdrawal was not due to new safety issues but was based upon the original evidence supplied to the CPMP and occurred as a result of due legal process. On 11 May 2001 the licenses were withdrawn for the second time. Subsequently, in November 2002, the European Court of Justice again overturned the original decision to ban anorectic drugs, including phentermine and amfepramone, and their licenses were once again reinstated.

At the current time, both phentermine and amfepramone are available. However, there seems little to support their continued use given the constraints on duration of treatment and the lack of long-term safety and efficacy evidence.

7.23 What results can we expect from using modern weight-loss drugs?

Studies with sibutramine and orlistat in a clinical setting have been designed to show what happens in 'real life'. Results from both are favourable, and indeed broadly comparable. On average, one can expect weight loss of around 9% maintained over 12 months, among those who respond to, and continue treatment. However, while every physician involved in weight management will be able to tell you of the marvellously successful patient who lost 40% body weight, they will equally be able to tell you of their abject failures.

SIBUTRAMINE

When used in conjunction with a low-calorie diet, data show that 77% of sibutramine-administered patients achieve a medically beneficial weight loss of at least 5% (James et al 2000). Importantly, continuation of therapy can sustain these weight losses for at least 2 years. Further, a recent meta-analysis has shown that, in sibutramine-administered obese patients, subjects who achieved weight losses of over 4 kg in the first 3 months of treatment were more likely to achieve long-term weight loss maintenance if therapy was continued. This in turn, led to marked improvements in metabolic factors such as lipid profile, insulin sensitivity and hypertension.

ORLISTAT

A placebo-controlled study (Sjostrom et al 1998) involving obese patients found that orlistat can promote and maintain weight loss (when administered in conjunction with a hypocaloric and a eucaloric diet, respectively). During the weight-loss phase (year 1), orlistat patients lost 10.2% body weight, compared with 6.1% in the placebo group. Results from the weight-maintenance phase of the trial (year 2) showed that patients who continued on orlistat regained half as much weight as patients switched to placebo. Weight-loss-associated improvements in cardiovascular risk factors, including lipid profile, blood pressure and fasting glucose, have also been demonstrated.

7.24 How do you choose which agent to use?

PATIENT PREFERENCE

Many patients will have heard of orlistat and/or sibutramine, from the press or from friends or family members, and will already have an informed, or sometimes ill-informed, preference. Some will not like the thought of a centrally acting agent influencing how they 'think' and will therefore be reluctant to consider sibutramine. Others will not take kindly to the risk of gastrointestinal side-effects of orlistat. It is important that the patient 'buys in' to whatever agent is chosen and therefore, perhaps more so than in other disease areas, patient preference is especially important.

CLINICAL CRITERIA

Both drugs are appropriate for use in patients with a BMI ≥30. Additionally, in the presence of serious comorbidities, orlistat can be used at a BMI ≥28 and sibutramine at a BMI ≥27. Each drug has a list of clinical contraindications and special precautions that will preclude them from use in some patients (*see Qs 7.9, 7.10, 7.14 and 7.15*).

It is vital that patients being considered for orlistat have adapted to a low-fat diet prior to treatment and all patients, whatever drug is chosen, must have demonstrated a commitment to long-term dietary and lifestyle change prior to commencement of treatment.

LIFESTYLE MODIFICATION RESPONSE

Orlistat is appropriate in those patients who have successfully adapted to a low-fat dietary regime. Sibutramine is appropriate for patients who have difficulty in maintaining modest portion sizes or avoiding snacks between meals. Clearly there will be cross-over here and neither drug is exclusive to any one type of patient.

7.25 Are the drugs expensive?

As with all medication, the cost has to be balanced against potential benefit to patients individually, and to society as a whole. Sibutramine and orlistat are not cheap and their use presents a significant challenge to NHS prescribing budgets. However, bearing in mind their short-term use (12 months) they compare very favourably to the cost of lifelong prescriptions of statins, glitazones, and other cardiovascular drugs:

■ Sibutramine costs approximately £35 for 28 days treatment: £455 for 1 year.
■ Orlistat costs approximately £41 for 28 days: £533 for 1 year.

NICE has produced favourable cost:benefit analyses of both agents.

7.26 For how long can they be used?

Unusually for drugs developed to tackle chronic illness, both orlistat and sibutramine have strict limitations imposed by their SPA licenses on their length of use:

■ Orlistat is licensed for use up to 24 months. NICE recommends that it is used for up to a maximum of 12 months normally and up to 24 months in exceptional circumstances.
■ Sibutramine is licensed for 12 months of treatment.

Available data suggest that many patients receive only 2 or 3 months of treatment. The probable explanation for this is likely to be unmet and unrealistic expectations – on the part of the patient or clinician. The rate of weight loss in the first few weeks is often too slow to satisfy a patient who has been struggling to lose weight for months, and possibly years. Other reasons might include poor pretreatment counselling – in the case of orlistat leading to perceived unacceptable GI side-effects, in the case of sibutramine to unpleasant but often transient dry mouth, headache or constipation.

The important thing is to use the drugs for as long as it takes, within the licensing regulations, to achieve the purpose for which they were started. After the initial weight-loss phase, drugs can play a crucial role in preventing weight regain, both prolonging the beneficial effects of weight loss and allowing more time for the patient to reinforce newly learned dietary and exercise habits.

7.27 What is the STORM trial?

The STORM study (Sibutramine Trial of Obesity Reduction and Maintenance) is a 2-year, double-blind, randomized, placebo-controlled multinational trial of sibutramine over 24 months. It showed significantly improved weight maintenance in those patients treated with sibutramine compared with those offered dietetic and lifestyle change support alone. A total of 605 obese patients (BMI 30–45) from eight European centres were included. All patients were treated for the initial 6 months with sibutramine 10 mg/day together with a low-fat, low-energy, individualized diet (600 kcal/day deficit) and exercise regimen. Of the 499 patients who completed the 6-month run-in period, 93% achieved >5% weight loss after 6 months and were randomized to either sibutramine 10 mg/day plus diet and exercise or placebo plus the same diet and exercise over a further 18 months. Those patients randomized to sibutramine were able to maintain their weight loss for up to 2 years: 43% of sibutramine patients who completed the trial maintained 80% or more of their original weight loss, compared with 16% of the placebo subjects (odds ratio 4.6, $P<0.001$). In addition, sibutramine-treated patients achieved beneficial improvements in a range of cardiovascular and metabolic parameters, such as HDL-cholesterol, VLDL-cholesterol, triglycerides, insulin and uric acid concentrations (*Fig. 7.1*).

7.28 What is XENDOS?

XENDOS (Xenical in the Prevention of Diabetes in Obese Subjects) was a multicentre study conducted in Sweden (Torgerson et al 2004). It treated obese people at risk of developing type 2 diabetes with orlistat over a 4-year period. A total of 3304 obese patients (BMI ≥30) with normal or impaired glucose tolerance were randomized to double-blind treatment with orlistat 120 mg or placebo tds in combination with a reduced-calorie diet and lifestyle modification.

At 4 years, the cumulative incidence rate of diabetes was significantly lower in the orlistat group than the placebo group (6.2% versus 9.0%), representing a 37.3% decrease with orlistat compared to placebo. Mean

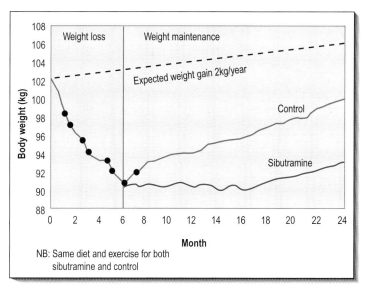

Fig. 7.1 STORM: mean bodyweight changes during weight-loss and weight-maintenance phases over 2 years (from James et al 2000, with permission from Elsevier).

TABLE 7.2 XENDOS results		
	Orlistat	Placebo
Mean weight loss (kg)		
1 year	11.4	7.5
4 years	6.9	4.1
Weight loss ≥5%		
1 year	79%	54%
4 years	53%	37%
Weight loss ≥10%		
1 year	45%	26%
4 years	26%	16%

weight loss was significantly greater in orlistat than placebo group at 1 year (*Table 7.2*). In addition, approximately 50% more orlistat-treated patients than placebo-treated patients achieved weight loss of ≥5% and ≥10%. Patients treated with orlistat also achieved a significantly greater reduction in waist circumference, a significantly greater improvement in

LDL-cholesterol and greater improvements in systolic and diastolic blood pressure than those who received placebo.

There continues to be a healthy debate over the use of medication to support weight maintenance far beyond the 12 months recommended use of both sibutramine and orlistat. In many patients, particularly those with active comorbidities, it can be argued that the benefits of continued weight maintenance are so great that the use of medication can be clinically justified. The issues against such prolonged use would be the licensing arrangements, the potential cost of long-term therapy and the effective acceptance of a failure to achieve sufficient long-term beneficial lifestyle change in that particular patient.

7.29 Can 'pulse therapy' be used?

There is little available data on the intermittent use, or 'pulse treatment', of weight-loss drugs. Most guidelines advocate a consistent use of medication for up to 12 months duration, during which time significant and long-term habit change is to be encouraged and supported. However, as our experience of modern weight-loss agents grows, it is apparent that many patients need clinical support long after a formal weight-loss programme. It would seem reasonable that where a patient remains highly motivated, and where the clinical risk supports it, repeated periods of drug treatment are justified to support weight maintenance and prevent the return or worsening of comorbid disease markers such as type 2 diabetes. Obesity is a chronic disease and even the most successful patients will require long-term support and intervention. It would seem short-sighted to withhold medication when the need is evident. This approach is not common in everyday practice but is likely to be increasingly seen in the years ahead as both the number of treated patients and general clinical experience increases.

7.30 Can drugs be used in combination?

Unlike hypotensive or hypoglycaemics agents, where the effect of using several drugs in combination produces an almost compound effect and has received universal acceptance, there is little evidence to support the simultaneous use of modern weight-loss drugs. Several studies have attempted to demonstrate the possible advantage of using sibutramine and orlistat in combination, but the data available to date suggest that there is only a slight advantage to be gained over using either of the drugs individually. The added cost of using two agents might make such an approach financially prohibitive.

7.31 Does prescribing one drug after another improve weight loss?

Very few studies have examined the potential benefits of prescribing one agent immediately after the cessation of another. The data that do exist suggest that there is little, if any, benefit to be gained. There might be a further slight reduction in weight but little clinical advantage is to be gained. The natural progress of any weight-loss programme is initial weight loss followed by a period of weight maintenance, and it would seem likely that, despite their very different modes of action, neither drug can radically alter this typical pattern of weight loss.

7.32 Is addiction or tolerance possible?

Agents such as phentermine are often said to produce amphetamine-like tolerance and addiction but there is little evidence to support this:

- Orlistat, because of its local mode of action, has no potential to give rise to chemical addiction.
- Despite its central mode of action and similarities with SSRI antidepressants, sibutramine shows no signs of addictive potential or subject misuse in preclinical trials and, since its launch, there have been no recorded cases of addiction.

However, all drugs used to aid weight loss must have some potential for psychological dependence, the patient fearing that weight maintenance without medication will prove too difficult to be sustainable, and lead to a return of weight lost. The importance of intensive lifestyle change support during treatment with medication cannot be stressed enough.

7.33 Can patients purchase drugs on the internet?

Numerous websites, some in the UK but many more overseas, are willing to supply prescription-only medications to a growing number of increasingly desperate overweight and obese patients. The dangers are self-evident. Cursory online health questionnaires, unsupported by clinical examination and reliant on patient-supplied information, can lead to inappropriate 'prescribing'. The lack of pretreatment counselling, the absence of a necessary follow-up examination and the risk of drug interactions, result in an intolerably high incidence of treatment side-effects, risk of serious complication to treatment and – inevitably – poor weight loss. Patients should always be discouraged from accessing weight loss medication in this manner.

7.34 What is the appropriate drug treatment for the comorbidities of obesity?

There are abundant guidelines governing the management of blood pressure and hypercholesterolaemia. These tell us exactly when to prescribe and what to offer our patients; they are beyond the scope of this book.

It is certainly appropriate to offer obese patients statins, ACE inhibitors, antihypertensives and aspirin, as dictated by their cardiovascular history. However, the potential weight gain caused by beta-blockers, and the cholesterol-raising effect of thiazides and beta-blockers should not be overlooked.

It should not be forgotten that specific pharmacotherapy for obesity is safe and effective, and reduces all the parameters associated with cardiovascular risk, although sibutramine is currently contraindicated if blood pressure is over 145/90 mmHg, and in the presence of a history of coronary heart disease.

UK-SPECIFIC QUESTIONS

7.35 What does NICE recommend?

The National Institute of Clinical Excellence (NICE) was formed in the UK to develop guidance for the NHS on the clinical- and cost-effectiveness of medical treatment, pharmacotherapy and surgical procedures.

In February 2001, NICE produced a report on orlistat (Xenical®); a report on sibutramine (Reductil®) followed in November 2001. Both reports recognized the high prevalence of obesity in the UK and the profound health consequences that result. They recommended the use of each medication only as an adjunct to medically supported lifestyle change programmes in patients with a BMI ≥30 or, in the presence of comorbidities, patients with a BMI ≥28 (orlistat) and BMI ≥27 (sibutramine). NICE also recommended that weight-management services be provided throughout the NHS to support the use of medication in both primary and secondary care.

7.36 Are the drugs available throughout the NHS?

The recommendations from NICE were given a mixed welcome by policy makers in primary care trusts (PCTs) and hospital trusts and, to date, the response has been very variable. The availability of orlistat and sibutramine within the NHS is in general widespread, but in some areas remains patchy. Some PCTs will not support the initiation of prescriptions for weight-loss medication from primary care but will accede to secondary care specialist recommendation. Other hospital trusts will not allow them to be included on hospital formularies but accept and support their use in primary care.

7.37 Why are some health authorities unwilling to fund drug treatment?

Despite the overwhelming evidence for the medical benefits of obesity management, and the efficacy and safety of modern medication, some decision makers seem unwilling to provide resources for obesity management. This is often due to fear of the costs that will result from the prescribing of medication. However, some are concerned about the lack of availability of skilled practitioners to deliver effective treatment in both primary and secondary care and a few remain sceptical about the likelihood of long-term weight loss, and so question the validity of treatment. Unfortunately, some are undoubtedly blinded by their own prejudice against obese patients, viewing the problem as self-inflicted and 'the patient's fault', and therefore not the responsibility of the NHS. In the National Service Framework (NSF) for coronary heart disease (CHD), published in the UK in February 2000, and in the NSF for diabetes (published in 2002), the Department of Health made clear its view that obesity management was integral to any future plans for the improved management of CHD and diabetes mellitus. Accordingly, each health authority was asked to develop and audit measures to combat overweight and obesity in its areas of influence.

7.38 Is there any additional patient support available?

The manufacturers of orlistat and sibutramine provide additional patient support materials:

■ Roche Products Ltd publishes the *Medical action plan* (MAP) and provides telephone dietetic and nursing advice for patients prescribed orlistat. Help is also available online for patients prescribed Xenical (http://www.xenicalmap.co.uk)

■ Abbott Laboratories Ltd provides the *Change for life* patient information and lifestyle modification programme to support those prescribed sibutramine and can also provide a professional's support pack for the prescriber (see http://www.changeforlifeonline.com).

Patients are given either a telephone number to call or information about the support programme when they receive their medication. There has been some concern that many patients prescribed medication do not use it for more than a few months at a time, so negating any significant benefit, and it is believed that the majority could be helped towards greater and long-term weight loss by using the additional support. About half of those prescribed orlistat or sibutramine make use of the programmes. In the authors' experience the majority of patients who use specifically designed support programmes find them helpful.

PATIENT QUESTIONS

7.39 Are the drugs addictive?

Orlistat acts locally in the gut to prevent the absorption of fat, and therefore has no potential to cause chemical addiction.

Despite its 'central' action, there is also no evidence, from clinical studies or experience, to suggest that sibutramine leads to dependency.

Older agents such as phentermine and other amfetamine-type drugs may lead to addiction because of their positive effect on mood. They have no place in a modern medical weight-loss programme.

7.40 Is there any risk of heart problems?

The combination drugs of fenfluoramine and phentermine, often called 'fen-phen', and of dexafenfluoramine and phentermine, was believed to cause valvular heart defects and was withdrawn from the European and US markets in 1997. Subsequent research has called into question these initial findings but their use remains controversial. There is no evidence to suggest that sibutramine causes cardiac valvular defects.

7.41 Will I still have to watch what I eat?

Absolutely. There is little to be gained by using medication alone without significant lifestyle change because weight loss will be minimal and very short term. In addition, the way orlistat works requires you to maintain a low-fat diet throughout treatment. Additionally, if you are not able to consciously modify your food intake during treatment you are not going to be able to maintain any weight loss in the long-term and will quickly regain weight. The time to change your dietary and exercise habits is now.

7.42 Will the weight stay off?

After weight loss, weight maintenance should be your goal. Using medication can help you to modify your dietary intake and lifestyle to lose weight and support you at the start of the weight-maintenance phase. However, in most cases their use is limited to 12 months. You should use the time on medication to help you to change your habits for good.

7.43 How long can I stay on the tablets?

You should expect to stay on treatment for at least 6 months, and for up to 12 months. Anything less than 6 months is likely to lead to short-term weight loss but not to significantly modified dietary and exercise habits. Although orlistat is licensed for use up to 24 months, it is recommended to be used for only up to 12 months, other than in 'exceptional circumstances'. Sibutramine can be used up to a maximum of 12 months.

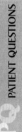

Management: surgery

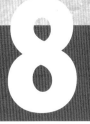

8

8.1 What are the methods of surgical treatment?

History is littered with unsuccessful procedures intended to cause weight loss:

No further surgical treatment of obesity has apparently been attempted since the tragical fate of a German Duke who in order to get leaner had the fat cut away by a Doctor in Upper Italy, and naturally succumbed to the operation (manuscript communication from Professor Dr DeLagarde 23 February 1882)

Other obsolete methods of surgery include jejunoileal bypass and jaw wiring, both of which are described later in this chapter.

There are two commonly used categories of bariatric surgery – restrictive and malabsorptive – and these are used either alone or in combination. More recently, implantable gastric pacing devices have been introduced.

8.2 Is there a place for surgery in modern management of obesity?

Surgical treatment of obesity is a vital facet of weight management and, in many, patients is the only effective method for losing weight. As in every other branch of surgery there have been massive technological advances in surgical procedures, resulting in safer, better and cheaper operations. The surgical option is limited to a few extremely obese people but for such patients it is an important means of significant long-term weight loss, and a huge improvement in health and quality of life.

8.3 What is bariatric surgery?

The term 'bariatric surgery' refers to surgical interventions and techniques that lead directly to weight loss and which are used for the treatment of obesity. The aim is to achieve the loss of around 50% of the excess body weight and to maintain weight loss in the long term.

8.4 How effective is bariatric surgery?

Bariatric surgery is an extremely successful long-term treatment for obesity. Because the surgical intervention is almost always permanent there is a much lower risk of rebound weight gain. Current procedures can be expected to induce a weight loss of, on average, 50–60% of excess body weight and a decrease in BMI of 10 kg/m^2 during the first 12–24 postoperative months (*Box 8.1*).

Mason et al (1997) studied 14 000 patients following various bariatric surgical procedures and found that they resulted in a mean loss of 53% of excess weight for vertical-banded gastroplasty and of 72% for gastric bypass.

BOX 8.1 The effect of bariatric surgery

After bariatric surgery, a person weighing 300 lb might realistically expect to achieve a weight of 200 lb; not 150 lb ('ideal body weight'). Most long-term studies show a modest weight gain (5–7 kg) after the initial postoperative period (Basiger et al 2000).

In the Swedish Obese Subjects (SOS) cohort study, which compared surgery (vertical-banded gastroplasty, gastric banding and gastric bypass) with conventional treatment, patients treated surgically had lost significantly more weight (on average 23%) after 2 years than patients managed conventionally, whose weight remained unchanged. This weight loss was maintained at 8 years and was equivalent to a difference in weight loss of 20.7 kg between those patients treated surgically and those managed conventionally (NICE 2002).

8.5 How many operations are done per year?

With the advent of laparoscopic gastric banding, surgery is becoming more common, as well as safer and cheaper, but there are still only a small number of procedures undertaken each year in the UK, where between 200 and 400 operations are carried out each year. More than half of these are funded privately. In the US, more than 70 000 operations are carried out every year.

8.6 What happens to markers of metabolic syndrome after bariatric surgery?

There are considerable improvements in comorbidities, including metabolic syndrome. Type 2 diabetes has been shown to resolve in 90% of patients, hypertension disappears in two-thirds, HDL can be seen to increase, and total cholesterol and triglycerides decrease. Cardiovascular parameters improve as well, including left ventricular wall thickness and left ventricular function. Pulmonary function improves and symptomatic sleep apnoea can disappear.

8.7 Who is eligible for bariatric surgery?

Bariatric surgery is normally recommended only for patients with a BMI of 40, or 35 with dangerous comorbidities. However, many surgeons would consider surgery to be an option in patients with a BMI of 35 in the absence of comorbidities if, for instance there is a poor family history of early mortality from heart disease or diabetes. Weight reduction surgery can only be considered for patients in whom non-surgical measures have failed.

8.8   What does NICE say about bariatric in the UK?

NICE has recommended the use of surgery 'when all other methods have failed', but has made it difficult for GPs to refer patients directly to a surgeon who will carry out the procedure. The guidelines insist that patients first undergo referral to specialist hospital clinics, and are submitted to a series of tests and multidisciplinary screening procedures that will probably already have been done by the GP. NICE guidance states:

Surgery is recommended as a treatment option for people with morbid obesity providing all of the following criteria are fulfilled:
- this type of surgery should be considered only for people who have been receiving intensive management in a specialized hospital obesity clinic
- individuals should be aged 18 years or over
- there should be evidence that all appropriate and available non-surgical measures have been adequately tried but have failed to maintain weight loss
- there should be no specific clinical or psychological contra-indications to this type of surgery
- individuals should be generally fit for anaesthesia and surgery
- individuals should understand the need for long-term follow-up.

8.9   How is 'morbid obesity' defined?

NICE defines morbid obesity 'for the purposes of the guidance' as:

A BMI either equal to or greater than 40 kg/m^2, or between 35 kg/m^2 and 40 kg/m^2 in the presence of significant comorbid conditions that could be improved by weight loss.

Other authorities use a broader definition. According to Balsiger et al (2000):

Patients have morbid obesity when they are 100% or greater above ideal body weight (IBW), are at least 100 lb above IBW or have a BMI of over 35. A strictly weight-based definition is not appropriate, however, and a better definition of morbid obesity includes patients who have direct, weight-related serious morbidity, such as mechanical arthropathy, hypertension, type 2 diabetes, lipid related cardiac disease, and sleep apnoea.

8.10   How many people suffer from morbid obesity?

In 1998, an estimated 0.6% of men and 1.9% of women in England and Wales had a BMI of 40 kg/m^2 or more – this is equivalent to 124 000 men and 412 700 women. People with a BMI >35 have a rate of mortality at any given age double that of someone with a BMI of 20–25.

8.11   How are patients selected for surgery?

Patients who undergo bariatric surgery will have initially presented to their doctor with concerns about their weight and have been given the appropriate advice relating to exercise, diet and lifestyle changes. They will often also have undergone pharmacotherapy. They will inevitably have been asked about their past medical history and previous attempts to lose weight, been examined and undergone screening investigations. The progression to considering surgery therefore indicates that these methods have not had the desired effect. NICE guidance insists that a hospital specialist at an obesity clinic must then be consulted, where a similar range of procedures will be carried out. Once under the care of a surgical team, patients will once again submit to a battery of questions and investigations before the operation can take place.

8.12 What importance do psychological factors have in the assessment for surgery?

There is a high prevalence of mental health conditions in grossly obese patients, including disordered eating, depression, low self-esteem and suicidal ideas. It is essential to diagnose and treat such conditions before embarking upon surgery, or to redirect patients to alternative channels of therapy. Postoperative problems often result from pre-existing depressive disorders not resolving as anticipated; such problems should be addressed beforehand.

The psychological implications of weight-loss surgery on an individual are immense. Patients undergo counselling to discuss their expectations of surgery, the reality of what they are actually letting themselves in for and are assessed as to whether they have the temperament and psychological stability to deal with the ramifications of surgery. Some patients are so desperate to lose weight at any cost that they do not give much thought to 'life after surgery'.

An individual takes a major step by surrendering control of his or her weight to another person. While undergoing conservative treatment, a patient can still choose whether to comply with the treatment or, for instance, to stray from dietary guidelines, to use the lift at work instead of walking up stairs, or not to renew a repeat prescription for their weight-loss pill. Their last voluntary act of weight management is to sign the consent form for surgery and submit to the anaesthetic. Thereafter, the surgeon assumes control and a permanent change takes place. After surgery, they will probably be physically unable to eat a meal above a certain size or to eat certain foods without discomfort. For some patients this handing over of responsibility amounts to an admission of failure, others view it as a great opportunity. Some individuals see it as a chance to deflect the blame onto someone else if they still don't lose weight.

There are profound changes in store for anyone undergoing weight-loss surgery. It is the duty of both the primary and secondary care teams to anticipate these changes and prepare individuals as thoroughly as possible beforehand, and to provide care and support – both physically and psychologically – after surgery. Patients will experience changes in body image and self-esteem, and changes in how they are viewed by their spouse, friends, relatives and the public. They might have problems coming to terms with the loss of freedom to eat and drink anything that takes their fancy; to go out and enjoy a meal without restriction and the possible unwanted side-effects of discomfort and vomiting

8.13 When is surgery contraindicated?

Some patients might decide not to opt for weight-loss surgery following screening, others might be deemed unsuitable; such patients should ideally be picked up in primary care.

The screening process might pick up biochemical evidence of an undiagnosed cause for obesity, or individuals for whom non-invasive management is clearly a better option. Patients might lose so much weight as a 'preoperative' measure that surgery is no longer necessary. In others there might be a psychological or underlying psychiatric condition that calls either for a different treatment altogether or needs to be dealt with before surgery is considered. Schizophrenia, personality disorder and uncontrolled depression are absolute contraindications for surgery. Individuals whose obesity is caused simply by love of food, or patients with binge eating disorder might find the postoperative adjustment of behaviour overwhelmingly difficult.

Prior to embarking on surgery, the risk:benefit ratio is considered and patients might be deemed unsuitable for surgery because of their comorbidities, anaesthetic risk and general well-being.

Women of childbearing age should be treated with extreme caution because of the increased nutritional needs of pregnancy being hampered by the reduced capacity for absorption of nutrients. Such patients are advised not to become pregnant after surgery until their weight has stabilized and their micronutrient status has been checked; contraceptive advice is essential.

8.14 What are the side-effects of surgery?

The most common side-effects of surgery are secondary to the small size of the stomach remnant in restrictive procedures, and include vomiting and the feelings of bloating and stomach distension. Malabsorptive procedures can lead to iron and vitamin B_{12} deficiency, and deficiency of other vitamins. Dumping syndrome is a relatively common occurrence. The complications of the obsolete jejunoileal bypass are potentially catastrophic and include acute hepatic failure, cirrhosis, oxalate nephropathy, chronic renal failure and malabsorption syndrome.

In the Danish Obesity Project and Swedish Obese Subjects (NICE 2002) trials, four deaths were directly attributable to surgical complications.

Perioperative problems included subphrenic abscess (7%), pneumonia (4%), wound infection (4–6%), pulmonary complications (3–6%) and hepatic dysfunction (1.5%).

Gallstones are a common long term side-effect.

8.15 What is the role of primary care?

Although some primary care professionals are well versed in the surgical management of obesity, many might not be well enough informed about the techniques and their ramifications to be able to offer adequate support to patients, and might know little about modern bariatric surgery techniques. Furthermore, because of the likely increase in the number of procedures being performed with the advent of laparoscopic techniques, coupled with the fact that surgical centres already have severely limited time for perioperative counselling, the GP's role is likely to assume greater significance. Primary care professionals should be knowledgeable enough to be able to give postoperative medium- and long-term support.

The GP is the first medical point of contact for patients who eventually undergo bariatric surgery, although only a small minority of a GP's patients will actually progress as far as surgery. The initial approach to the topic of weight-loss surgery is likely to be through primary care and the GP should be aware of the various operative techniques and their side-effects, with special emphasis on the permanent nature of such procedures.

Every potential candidate for surgery will have undergone first-line treatment by diet, lifestyle changes, behavioural therapy and usually drug therapy by the time he or she is ready to discuss surgery, and a GP should ideally be aware which patients are suitable for surgery and what the operative criteria are. The GP should convey to a patient the realistic expectations of weight loss surgery; for instance, that they will probably lose about 50% of their excess weight but might still consider themselves overweight once their condition stabilizes.

It is usual for patients to undergo multidisciplinary screening in hospital prior to undergoing surgery; each individual is given a thorough medical and psychological assessment to ascertain suitability for the procedure. Most patients will already have been investigated in primary care or hospital obesity clinics, but will have further biochemical and metabolic screening carried out, as well as sleep studies if appropriate.

8.16 What is meant by restrictive surgery?

Restrictive surgery reduces the size of the stomach so than less food can be ingested before a feeling of fullness occurs. If any more food is eaten it can result in bloatedness and will be regurgitated or vomited. Examples of restrictive surgery include gastric stapling and laparoscopic gastric banding. Once food has passed through the restricted portion of the stomach it will pass normally through the rest of the bowel, so that nutrients will be absorbed normally.

8.17 What is meant by malabsorptive surgery?

Malabsorptive surgery reduces the length of bowel through which the food passes, so that a smaller amount will be adsorbed. Patients can therefore eat what they want but pass unabsorbed nutrients through the bowel. Examples are shown in *Fig. 8.1*, and include Roux-en-Y bypass and jejunoileal bypass.

8.18 What are implantable gastric stimulation devices?

Gastric stimulation is a recently developed approach to surgically induced weight loss. A small laparoscopically implanted pacing device – an implantable gastric stimulation (IGS) device, developed from an original concept by Dr Valerio Cigaina in Italy – provides electrical stimulation to the smooth muscle of the wall of the stomach. The IGS is placed in a subcutaneous pocket in the abdomen. Surgery usually takes less than 1 hour. An external programmer communicates non-invasively with the implanted device and allows modification of the electrical parameters. The gastric stimulation produces an increase in satiety levels and results in decreased calorific intake. It can therefore help patients lose weight in combination with standard behaviour and dietary modifications. Early studies in Europe and North America in over 200 patients show weight loss equating to 25% of excess body weight after 3 years, with a remarkably low level of immediate postoperative and long-term adverse complications. Advantages would appear to be the ease of surgical insertion, the relative absence of side-effects and the very promising long-term results. Disadvantages include the battery life of the pacer (average 5 years) and the possible future need for replacement.

8.19 What is a jejunoileal bypass?

This procedure is no longer performed. More than 90% of the small bowel was bypassed by attaching the beginning of the jejunum to the end of the ileum, leaving a total of only 18 functional inches. This caused rapid transit of food through the bowel and incomplete digestion, leading to malabsorption and severe steatorrhoea. The aim was to allow subjects to eat an unrestricted diet with no change in eating habits, and still lose weight. Although successful in that respect, it caused an unacceptable incidence of severe, occasionally life-threatening complications and side-effects, including acute hepatic failure, cirrhosis, oxalate nephropathy and chronic renal failure, immune complex arthritis and malabsorption syndromes. Although this procedure was abandoned around 1980, patients with late side-effects are occasionally encountered in primary care.

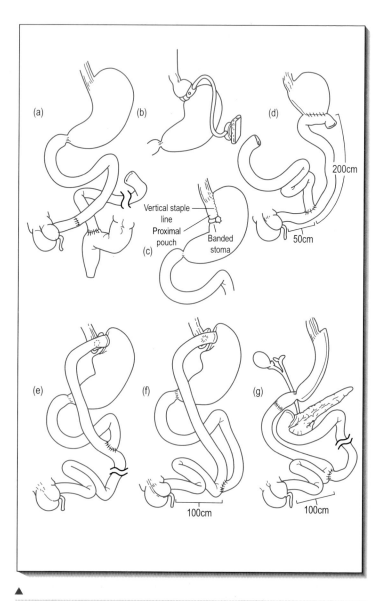

▲

Fig. 8.1 Past and current bariatric operations. (a) Jejunoileal bypass, (b) gastric banding, (c) vertical-banded gastroplasty, (d) partial biliopancreatic bypass, (e) Roux-en-Y gastric bypass, (f) very, very long limb Roux-en-Y gastric bypass, (g) partial biliopancreatic bypass with duodenal switch.

8.20 What is a gastroplasty?

The word literally means 'changing the shape of the stomach'. This is performed by partitioning a pouch of between 15 and 40 mL at the top of the stomach. This fills rapidly with food and empties slowly, through a narrow channel, into the body of the stomach. The pouch restricts the volume of food a person can eat by reducing the stomach's functional capacity. Among the most commonly used procedures is the vertical-banded gastroplasty.

Laparoscopic gastric banding involves wrapping an adjustable band around the outside of the stomach to prevent distension and restrict intake. The degree of restriction is altered by increasing or decreasing the pressure through an epigastric or abdominal port.

8.21 What are the advantages and disadvantages of restrictive surgical procedures?

The restrictive procedures have the advantages of technical ease, low morbidity, lack of any malabsorption (as food eventually passes through the gastrointestinal tract in the usual way) and lower cost. However, the degree of sustained weight loss might not be as great as in other procedures. Also, some patients recognize that high-calorie liquids such as milkshakes, ice-cream and alcohol pass rapidly through the stoma without causing fullness, and change their diet accordingly, thereby regaining weight.

8.22 What is a gastric bypass?

Gastric bypass surgery, or Roux-en-Y bypass is widely used as a first-line procedure. A 10-mL segment is isolated from the body of the stomach, surgically separated from the remainder of the organ and anastomosed to the proximal jejunum, bypassing most of the stomach and the entire duodenum. This has the advantage of restricting intake in the same way as gastroplasty, as well as inducing a degree of malabsorption. The advantage of gastric bypass surgery is that it is thought to be more effective in inducing and maintaining long-term weight loss because of its double action. The disadvantages are that it is a bigger and more technically demanding operation than the gastroplasty, and that malabsorption, in particular of iron, folate and vitamin B_{12} can occur postoperatively, requiring careful monitoring for life.

8.23 What forms of surgery are available for patients whose obesity is immediately life threatening?

Specialist forms of surgery have been designed for 'superobese' individuals with a BMI >50, 225% overweight or weighing more than 400 lb with life-threatening, obesity-related morbidity. These involve 80% distal gastrectomy and gastroileostomy with diversion of biliary and pancreatic secretions to the distal ileum. This is said to result in intense weight loss with malabsorption, especially of the fat-soluble vitamins, folate, vitamin B_{12}, iron and calcium, all of which need monitoring and, if necessary, supplementing.

8.24 What is the role of liposuction?

Liposuction involves the suction of fatty material from under the skin by way of a trochar. It usually results in the removal of approximately 3 L of fat, but can sometimes involve the loss of 10–12 L in extreme cases. Although the technique has been attempted as a treatment for the morbidly obese, its value is as a cosmetic procedure. It has no influence on visceral or abdominal adiposity and therefore has no appreciable physiological effects on insulin resistance or other comorbid disease markers.

8.25 What is the role of jaw wiring?

Jaw-wiring procedures are no longer recommended. The weight lost was rapidly regained once the wires were removed, often despite the fitting of a cord round the waist to limit the amount of weight regained.

8.26 What is the purpose of apronectomy?

Apronectomy is not a treatment for obesity but is helpful for patients who have lost large quantities of weight and have overhanging folds of excess skin. Skin contouring operations are not restricted to the abdomen; other sites include brachioplasty, and the inner and outer aspects of the thighs. Abdominal apronectomy can be circumferential, and males can undergo gynaecomastia correction.

It can be very psychologically damaging to deny patients such surgery on cost or other grounds after they have followed medical advice diligently but are left feeling uglier and with a lower self-esteem than when they started. It is a technically straightforward procedure, and its satisfying results can help maintain long-term weight loss.

8.27 What is an artificial bezoar?

An artificial bezoar is a balloon or other object that is inserted into the stomach to lessen its capacity as a restrictive technique. It has a limited role but can be beneficial in, for instance, initiating weight loss in the short term in individuals who are not fit for more major surgical procedures.

8.28 What are the costs of bariatric surgery?

The average cost of surgical intervention is between £5300 and £13 000 but these figures will reduce markedly with the increase in laparoscopic techniques. Operations are carried out either by specialist bariatric surgeons – a rare breed in the UK – or, more commonly, by GI surgeons with an interest in antiobesity surgery.

8.29 What is the general surgical risk associated with obesity?

Obesity, especially morbid obesity, adds significantly to perioperative risk. A Canadian study (Chung et al 1999) revealed that obese patients were four times more likely to develop perioperative respiratory events, whereas a separate study (Eichenberger et al 2002) revealed that, in the morbidly obese, adverse respiratory events were linked with increased levels of pulmonary atelectasis during anaesthesia. It has been suggested that postoperative continuous positive airways pressure might prevent this.

Extra care is needed to calculate drug dosages in obese patients because renal clearance of drugs is increased with raised renal blood flow and glomerular filtration rate, and also because drugs such as benzodiazepines and barbiturates are highly lipophilic (Ogunnaike et al 2002).

Preoperative assessment of the obese patient includes evaluation for systemic and pulmonary hypertension, right and left ventricular failure and ischaemic heart disease. Methods include echocardiography, ECG, chest X-ray and, in extreme cases, pulmonary artery catheterization. Blood gases might detect CO_2 retention and hypoxia before or during surgery. Peripheral and central access can be hampered by excess fat at cannulation sites and intubation might be hazardous because of excess cervical fat and palatal and pharyngeal soft tissue; the patient's neck might need to be 'stacked' by placing towels or blankets beneath it.

Antibiotic prophylaxis is commonly given to obese patients because of the increased risk of skin infections. The risk of aspiration pneumonitis is reduced by H_2-antagonists or proton pump inhibitors. Morbid obesity is a major risk factor for sudden death from postoperative pulmonary embolism; perioperative heparin reduces the risk of this, and also of deep vein thrombosis. Opioids are avoided if possible because of respiratory depression, and intramuscular and subcutaneous routes are avoided because of unreliable absorption.

Regular operating tables have a maximum weight limit of 205 kg; extra large tables can cope with up to 455 kg although often two tables are put together for superobese patients. In any case, it is important to protect pressure areas because pressure ulcers and neural injuries are particularly common in obese patients.

PATIENT QUESTIONS

8.30 Is weight-loss surgery a good idea?

Weight-loss surgery is an extremely effective way of losing weight, and keeping the weight off. These days it is remarkably safe and straightforward, with very few risks. But having an operation to lose weight will alter a person's life permanently and he or she will no longer be able to eat more than a few mouthfuls of soft food at a time without feeling bloated or sick, so going out for dinner or entertaining friends becomes an entirely different proposition after surgery. A person might well lose an enormous amount of weight after an operation, and will look entirely different to family and friends. He or she might feel able to do more and be more physically active. It is important for someone considering surgery to spend time planning ahead to try to foresee any pitfalls to ensure that surgery is the correct option.

Obesity in children

PQ PATIENT QUESTIONS

9.1 What is the prevalence of overweight and obesity in children?

Just as in adults, the past 30 years have seen a rapid escalation in the prevalence of overweight and obesity in children, to the extent that it is now the most common metabolic disorder affecting children. Across Europe there are comparable increases to be seen among boys and girls but within each nation the prevalence rate varies considerably. Recent figures for the Netherlands put the number of overweight children, corresponding to an adult with a BMI of greater than 25, at 7% but in Malta the rate is 55%. In the UK, between 1989 and 1998, the prevalence of overweight in children under the age of 5 years increased from 14.7 to 23.6% and the prevalence of obesity from 5.4 to 9.2%. Similar findings have been reported between 1974 and 1994 in the UK in older children, with levels of overweight rising from 8 to 13% in girls.

As children become older, the overall prevalence of overweight and obesity increases. In 1999, prevalence rates in the UK for overweight and obesity ranged from 22% at age 6 years, 23% at 10, 26% at 13 to as much as 30% at 15 years. The prevalence of obesity rose in a similar fashion from 10% at 6 years to 15% at age 15.

9.2 What are the risks to obese children?

Children who are overweight and obese carry very similar risks to those experienced in adults. Among obese adolescents, one-third carry one additional risk factor for comorbid disease and as much as another one-third carry two additional risk markers.

The most common comorbid diseases are hypertension, dyslipidaemia, type 2 diabetes, sleep apnoea and orthopaedic problems such as slipped femoral epiphysis. Obese children also have a predisposition to Blount's disease of the tibia (tibia vara). There are also well-researched and identified problems of low self-esteem, bullying at school, psychological illness and eating disorders. Type 2 diabetes, once called 'maturity onset diabetes' and restricted mainly to those in middle age and above, is being increasingly identified in obese teenagers.

Such is the problem of type 2 diabetes in children in some parts of the US that in some centres one-third of Afro-American and Caucasian children who have diabetes have been identified as type 2 diabetics. In 1999, one UK specialist paediatric clinic was unaware of any children with type 2 diabetes. By 2001, of 300 diabetic children under its care, 11 were identified as having type 2 diabetes related to obesity. Further reports from the same specialist clinic reveal an incidence among obese children who attend the clinic of 60% for systolic hypertension and 62% of significant dyslipidaema.

As many as 28% of adolescents attending the clinic were thought to have metabolic syndrome, as defined by the WHO.

In 2002, Sinha et al reported that in children of between 4 and 10 years of age with a BMI greater than the 95th centile, 25% had evidence of impaired glucose tolerance and 4% had frank type 2 diabetes. Also in 2002, Sorof and Daniels reported an increased prevalence of hypertension in overweight children with a BMI greater than the 95th centile, with more than 25% being hypertensive.

Up to 75% of obese children go on to become obese adults, carrying with them the same risk factors for comorbid disease into adulthood. It is recognized that weight gain during childhood is a risk factor for adult cardiovascular disease. Direct correlations have been made between weight and BMI during childhood and adult levels of fasting insulin, lipids and systolic blood pressure.

9.3 Do obese children develop insulin resistance?

Just as in adults, obesity in children can lead to increased insulin resistance. Obesity, hypertension, dyslipidaemia and impaired glucose tolerance are common features. The ATP III definition of the metabolic syndrome can be found on page 40, Q 3.14.

9.4 What causes obesity in children?

Children are ultimately subject to the same genetic and environmental influences as adults. It is no surprise, therefore, that we have seen increases in prevalence rates mirroring those of adults over the past 30 years. The presence of a parental history of obesity among obese and non-obese children under 10 years of age doubles the risk of a child being obese as an adult. Studies of identical twins suggest that inherited predisposition might be as high as 75%.

Three key life events seem to be associated with the development of childhood obesity:

- the prenatal period
- the period of adiposity rebound
- adolescence.

These are discussed in detail in *Box 9.1*.

Environmental change over the past 30 years is clearly associated with the development of obesity in children but to date it has not been possible to provide direct causative links. Prentice & Jebb (1995) showed quite clearly the association between increased TV viewing and availability of private cars with the rise in obesity. Other studies have shown an association between the availability of high-fat, high-sugar foods and obesity development. It is widely recognized that a decrease in formal physical activity in the school

---

BOX 9.1 Major events associated with obesity in children

The prenatal period

A high birthweight appears to be associated with a high risk of childhood obesity. Infants of diabetic mothers are also at particular risk, and may therefore have made interpretation of these results difficult. A high birthweight may affect subsequent development of obesity because of physiological programming occurring due to the prenatal experience, and might involve influences on hypothalamic set points for bodyweight due to the effects of above average intrauterine nutrition.

Adiposity rebound

This describes the increase in BMI that follows the lowest point in BMI that occurs prior to the age of 5 years. Between the years of 5 and 6, the BMI begins to rise and continues to do so throughout childhood and into early adulthood. This 'rebound' can serve as a predictor of the likelihood of adult obesity; the earlier the rebound occurs, the more likely the child is to have a high BMI in adulthood.

Adolescence

The third and greatest period of risk is in adolescence. Up to 75% of obesity present in adolescence persists into adulthood, and carries at least the same, if not greater, risk for the development of comorbid disease in adulthood, including cardiovascular disease, diabetes, colorectal cancer, gout and osteoarthritis. Early pubertal maturation appears to increase the risk of adult obesity.

---

playground, a perception of increased danger in walking to school and the development of computer games consoles have led to an overall decrease in physical activity in children. A child spending 1 hour watching TV expends less energy than 1 hour reading a book. One study showed that children watching 4 or more hours of TV daily were eight times more likely to be overweight than children watching half as much TV. The risk of overweight in young teenagers increases by 2% for every extra hour of TV viewing per week.

Simultaneously, social trends towards families where both parents work has led to a deterioration in many aspects associated with family life, including family mealtimes, home-prepared food and an increase in high-fat, high-sugar snacks, both at school and at home. The consumption of sugary drinks has increased, as has the individual portion size of each drink. The aggressive marketing of such products undoubtedly has a role to play in this but is not the sole reason for the development of childhood obesity. As children become overweight they are less inclined to engage in physical activity, which only compounds the problem. Lack of participation in active play can result in social isolation and withdrawal. This can in turn lead to a lowering of self-esteem, comfort eating and, on occasions, eating disorders.

9.5 What is wrong with the average child's diet?

The increase in availability and acceptance of high-fat, high-sugar foods has undoubtedly contributed to the increased development of obesity. Fast food and take-away food is usually cheap, convenient and palatable. It is also high in fat and sugar. For decades, aggressive marketing campaigns to promote the consumption of such foods have associated them with images of happiness, contentment and fun. Millions of people are now convinced that 'happiness' comes in the form of a small but calorie-charged children's fast-food meal.

The advertising of such high-fat, high-sugar foods has caused a great deal of concern throughout Europe and internationally. It is thought that as much as 80–90% of advertising that takes place during peak children's TV viewing hours promotes the consumption of high-fat, high-sugar foods. Many concerned organizations have raised the issue with national governments. In the UK at the time of writing (2004), the government position is that such advertising does not influence total consumption but rather influences brand choice. The same argument has been used to defend the advertising of cigarettes and tobacco products; few are convinced by this stance.

It is not only the frequency of eating such foods that has changed, even portion sizes have increased. Between 1970 and 1996, the average salty snack has risen in calorific value by 93 kcal, or 60%. Soft drinks, once an occasional 90-kcal treat, now pack an extra 49 kcal per sugar-loaded can. Fast-food servings of fries, and the calorie content of burgers, have increased by 20%. It is hard for children to resist 'supersizing' their fast-food meals when this is offered at so little extra cost. These increases have also led to increased sizes of serving plates in restaurants and have been mirrored in portion sizes inside the home.

9.6 How much energy do children expend?

There has been a gradual decrease in children's physical activity levels over the past few decades. In 2000, a UK government survey found that 40% of boys and 60% of girls were failing to engage in physical activity of moderate intensity for at least 1 hour each day. The amount of PE in schools has decreased gradually over the past 20 years and children's hobbies have become much more sedentary. Formal play has diminished and fears about the safety of the roads because of increasingly busy traffic and highly publicized child abduction cases have resulted in the majority of children being driven to school.

There is little evidence to *prove* the association between the development of childhood obesity and the decrease in physical activity but the evidence would appear to be staring us in the face. Some research has shown that decreases in weight are associated with increases in lifestyle exercise, for example walking to activities, using stairs whenever possible, and decreased TV viewing and computer use.

9.7 How do we manage obesity in children?

Managing overweight and obesity in children requires sensitivity, patience, understanding and the application of different techniques to those employed in adulthood. The same basic principles apply but the application must be modified to make them appropriate to children.

In 2002 the Royal College of Paediatrics and Child Health and the National Obesity Forum published the first guidelines for professionals for the management of overweight in children and adolescents. The guidelines were designed to be succinct, with clear practical applications. They were not designed to provide all the answers but rather to assist clinicians to work with the majority of their patients. Other guidelines have since been developed and, at the time or writing, the Scottish Intercollegiate Guidelines Network (SIGN) is developing more substantial guidelines.

9.8 Who should be involved in managing overweight in children?

As in adult weight management, all members of the clinical team have a role to play. The physician might be the first to identify the problem, a parent might bring a child to the physician for advice on weight management or the nurse might be the first professional presented with a request for assistance. It might fall upon teachers to notice the development of obesity in a pupil and a referral could come through a school nurse or a health visitor. Within the secondary care sector, specialist paediatricians work with specialist dieticians and paediatric nurses, and often also with community paediatricians and clinical psychologists, to deliver a comprehensive team approach. What is important is that the child trusts these professionals and can develop a rapport with them. It might be appropriate for the professional in whom the child has most confidence to lead the weight management programme.

9.9 How is obesity in children defined?

The standard measure of obesity in children remains the BMI, calculated by taking the child's weight in kilograms and dividing it by their height in metres squared (*see Chapter 1*). The BMI fluctuates throughout childhood and therefore is not in isolation directly applicable to the assessment of overweight in children. In 1997 the International Obesity task force agreed an international standard for BMI centile charts. It was agreed by a panel of experts that the most appropriate way to establish criteria for overweight and obesity was to correlate the BMI centiles with a BMI of ≥25 and ≥30 in 18-year-olds, and to extend them to identify overweight and obesity in younger children. These diagnostic thresholds approximate the 85th and 95th centiles and should be regarded as the levels of BMI at which a child is to be viewed as being overweight and obese respectively. In the US, some clinicians, concerned about the negative effects of terminology on adolescents, refer to the 95th centile as 'overweight' and the 85th centile as being the threshold to define those 'at risk of overweight'. Whatever the terminology, the same disease risk rates apply at the 85th centile and the 95th centile. There is as yet no agreement on what might constitute morbid obesity in children.

Waist circumference is not normally used in assessing obesity in children; it has not been shown to correspond to the same disease risk ratios as BMI as it has in adults. Similarly, body fat mass does not seem to correspond directly to the BMI centiles and is not generally used. However, it might be appropriate to use body fat mass assessment as a means of engaging a child who might otherwise be reluctant to stand on scales and have their BMI calculated. A salutatory lesson is to be learned: engaging an overweight or obese child in a programme will require more tact and creativity than that normally employed for adults. BMI centile charts can be bought in the UK from Harlow Printing (Maxwell Street, South Shields, Tyne and Wear, NE53 4PU; http://www.health-for-all-children.co.uk/acatalog).

The decision to intervene in the management of a child whom you suspect of being overweight must depend upon the degree of overweight, the child's age, the presence of any psychological or physical comorbidity and the level of commitment – from both the child and the family – in considering significant long-term lifestyle change. Involving the whole family is essential because it is highly unlikely that a child will be able to modify dietary and activity habits in the absence of positive support from his or her carers.

9.10 How do you assess an obese child?

When making an assessment of the best way to approach weight loss in a child, several considerations must be made:

- Why is help being requested?
- Is the child him-/herself concerned or is the family pressurizing the child to seek help?
- Is there a family history of obesity-related disease? (this would lower the threshold for intervention)

An assessment of physical activity levels and eating patterns needs to be made; keeping a food diary (*see Q 6.36*) might be helpful but parental support for this would be essential. A balance must be struck between helping the child become more aware of poor eating habits in order to promote healthier choices, and making the child too focused on calorie counting and food watching.

When taking a history of eating patterns it is important to consider the presence of eating disorders. Such disorders include binge eating disorder (*see Q 4.10*), comfort eating, night eating syndrome (*see Q 4.11*) or self-induced vomiting. Other behavioural abnormalities include the use of laxatives to promote weight loss.

An observation of the child's psychological state (and that of the parents) must be made, looking at psychological reasons both as a possible cause for overweight and as a possible effect. An assessment of the child's academic progress is also important. Obesity can reduce the likelihood of academic success. Similarly, a child who is intellectually challenged can present increasingly difficult clinical problems.

9.11 What examination is necessary?

A physical examination of an overweight child is advisable but not strictly necessary. If a child is embarrassed to be weighed it might be better to delay physical assessment until he or she has gained more confidence. Ideally, one would conduct measurements of height, weight and BMI with reference to centile charts. An examination for features of congenital or endocrine disease should be made and, if acceptable to the child, an appropriate evaluation of pubertal development. Blood pressure (using an appropriate-sized cuff) and urine analysis for glucose and protein are desirable. Further investigations might be indicated if there is evidence of short stature, dysmorphic features, learning disability and no obvious family history of obesity.

9.12 What rare causes of obesity exist?

The vast majority of children are obese because of environmental influences superimposed on their genetic predisposition. However, it is imperative that the clinician is aware of, and seeks out, rare causes of obesity such as endocrine disease (including hypothyroidism, Cushing's syndrome and growth hormone deficiency). Some children are obese because of prescribed medication, for example corticosteroids in a chronic asthmatic. There are also very rare chromosome abnormalities such as Prader–Willi syndrome, a single gene defect that causes leptin deficiency. The condition is characterized by voracious appetite: the child eats huge amounts of food and appears to be insatiable. The level of obesity is extremely severe at a very early age. Suspicion of the Prader–Willi syndrome requires referral for specialist assessment (*see Q 2.15*). Other factors that need to be considered are predisposing factors for obesity such as spina bifida, muscular dystrophy and other causes of immobility, and PCOS.

9.13 When should specialist help be requested?

Referral to a specialist paediatrician should be considered in the presence of serious comorbidities such as type 2 diabetes, hypertension or sleep apnoea. Also consider referral if the child:

- is of low stature (below the 9th centile or relative to the immediate family)
- has developed precocious puberty (before 8 years)
- has developed late puberty (after 13 years).

Note: there are gender differences for the ages of onset of precocious and late puberty; please refer to the guidelines (see http://www.national obesityforum.org.uk).

The presence of a significant learning disability and any signs of genetic or endocrine abnormality would make specialist involvement essential.

Severe progressive obesity under the age of 2 years requires further specialist investigation.

Drug therapy is not commonly used in the management of childhood overweight and, although it can be considered as a possible option, particularly in adolescents, primary care clinicians would be advised to seek specialist advice.

9.14 What weight-loss goals should be set?

In determining what weight-management goals should be set, the following criteria should be considered:

- No weight gain as the height increases (therefore the BMI decreases).
- Weight gain slower than height gain.
- Rapid weight loss is inappropriate except under specialist care.
- In exceptional circumstances, in children over 7 years of age suffering from obesity and in the presence of comorbid disease, weight loss of 0.5 kg per month might be acceptable.
- In adolescence (fully grown) 0.5-kg weight loss per week might be appropriate.

Parental and family involvement is essential.

9.15 What dietary interventions should be advised?

Some specialists advocate calculating the daily calorific requirements of a child and making specifically calculated calorific reductions. However, this specialist expertise is not readily available to the vast majority of clinicians and the approach outlined in *Box 9.2* is therefore more appropriate.

BOX 9.2 Recommendations for dietary intervention in childhood obesity

The initial aim should be to return the child to a normal, healthy daily eating pattern. Aim for a balanced varied meal, not just for the child but also for the rest of the family:

- Encourage the child to have three meals a day, starting with breakfast, and to avoid eating between meals, 'grazing' and definitely to avoid TV dinners.
- Encourage the parents not to use food or snacks as rewards for good behaviour but, where recognition of good behaviour is required, to use fruit as an alternative.
- Encourage a move towards less energy-dense foods and, except for children under 7 years of age, towards low-fat alternatives.
- Encourage the inclusion of wholefoods, which are more likely to lead to satiety, in the diet. Fruit and wholemeal bread should be encouraged, as should a minimum of five portions of fruit and vegetables each day. As a guide, a 'portion' of fruit or vegetables is equivalent to the amount a child can hold in his or her hand.
- Fizzy drinks should be limited and, when chosen, should always be low calorie or 'diet' drinks.

It is important that the child is not forced to embrace any kind of 'diet' because this can result in disillusionment and rejection. Mealtimes should remain fun and enjoyable and should be a family occasion as often as possible. It is important not to isolate the child from his or her siblings and peers.

9.16 What makes up a portion of fruit and vegetables?

A portion of fruit and vegetables is the amount the child can hold in his or her hand. Specific examples are given in *Box 9.3*.

9.17 What physical activity advice should be given?

In 2000, a UK government survey found that 40% of boys and 60% of girls were failing to engage in physical activity of moderate intensity for at least 1 hour a day. Any increase in physical activity levels will therefore help.

Parents are not likely to be able to influence activities during the school day, where obese children are noticeably less active than their normal-weight counterparts, but they can greatly influence activity at home. Obese children tend to be late risers, especially on weekend mornings. Encouragement to get up earlier, spend less time watching TV during the day and gentle encouragement towards formalized exercise might help.

BOX 9.3 Fruit and vegetable portions for a child

Fruit
- 1 small apple, pear or banana
- 12 grapes
- small orange or a plum
- one glass of fruit juice (250 mL)

Vegetables
- 2 tablespoons peas or sweetcorn
- 2 small carrots
- 4 small tomatoes

Note: Fruit juice can count only once, and potatoes don't count at all, although baked beans do.

Parents could place a limit on TV and computer use to say, perhaps, 1 hour a day. For others, family walks and cycling can help.

The parents should be encouraged to make time to walk the child to and from school, to work out safe routes to walk to friends' houses or to the park, and to encourage the child constantly. They might choose to set a goal that all journeys of less than 1 km will be made on foot. Above all, activity needs to be enjoyable, have purpose and be sustainable; it must never be embarrassing. Within the school day, contact with a motivated teacher who understands the child's need for increased activity can help in encouraging the child to become more active, ensuring participation in PE lessons, extracurricular activities and sport.

An overweight child might have gradually withdrawn from formal exercise at school and a gradual reintroduction is essential. It is difficult to quantify just how much activity is required. A sustainable increase of any amount can be beneficial, both in terms of weight management and self-esteem.

9.18 What long-term management goals should be set?

All goals should be small, reasonable, achievable and sustainable. When possible, they should be agreed with the child and his or her parents. Some adolescents might choose to attempt weight management without parental interference, and this should be recognized and respected. If problems with teasing and bullying have been identified, coping strategies need to be developed and these might involve teachers and the school authorities, not just health professionals.

Any identified psychosocial issues need to be addressed. Involvement of specialist counsellors might be an advantage in offering extra support and expertise.

One aim should be the development of positive parenting skills. Helping parents to deal with disordered eating and behavioural difficulties is never easy. The involvement of health visitors, even with the families of older children, should be considered. Aim to see the child regularly. Ideally, initial appointments should be weekly or 2-weekly. The frequency can reduce as confidence grows and treatment strategies develop but, at a minimum, monthly appointments must be offered.

9.19 What is successful weight management in children?

Success can be measured in many ways. For young children, weight maintenance – keeping the weight static as they grow taller – leads to a reduction in BMI and might be sufficient. For older children, over 7 years old, sustained weight loss of 0.5 kg per month over a period of time would be a huge success. For fully-grown adolescents, repeated weight loss of 0.5 kg per week is a major achievement.

In addition to weight maintenance or weight loss, success must be measured in terms of improved dietary health and activity levels, improvements of which, even in the absence of weight change, can lead to significantly improved general health and reduction in disease risk. The general well-being of the child, enhanced self-esteem, more contentment and peer-acceptability at school, and improved family dynamics are also very significant areas in which success can be measured, and achieved.

9.20 How long should follow-up last?

The child (and the parents) might reach a stage where they feel satisfied with progress made (or, alternatively, disillusioned by lack of progress) and cease regular contact. This does not necessarily mean that they have given up. They might have decided to pursue weight management on their own, often using the techniques and strategies previously offered. The nature of weight management, in adults and children, is that motivation to succeed, drive and adherence to what can appear to be draconian treatment principles will fluctuate wildly, even on a daily basis.

Obesity is not a curable disease and more than half of obese adolescents go on to become obese adults. Even in 'successful' cases, where weight loss has been marked, the propensity to regain weight is highly likely to remain and relapses are common. The clinician should remain open to renewed requests for support, either as occasional advice or more intense treatment plans.

9.21 Is there a role for weight-loss drugs in children?

The very thought of using drugs to induce weight loss in children will initially be an anathema to most clinicians. However, when we consider that in some children we are dealing with a serious, life-

> threatening disease process, if lifestyle interventions fail, is it fair to withhold effective medications? After all, we would not flinch at treating their type 2 diabetes with drugs, so shouldn't we also treat their obesity? The moral arguments are likely to continue for some time.

Research is being done to assess the applicability, efficacy and safety of using the modern weight loss drugs orlistat and sibutramine in adolescents (*see Chapter 7*). One such study, using orlistat 120 mg tds for 3 months in 20 teenagers whose average age was 14 years, found that an average weight loss of 3.6% could be achieved, with comparative reductions in body fat composition, BMI, lipid levels and waist circumference. Side-effects similar to those in adults were experienced. Vitamin D deficiency was observed in three cases, all of whom had low levels of vitamin D prior to treatment. Similar studies are also being conducted using sibutramine. It would appear that, in short-term studies at least, medication can positively influence weight loss outcome in adolescents. It should be noted that neither orlistat nor sibutramine are promoted or even licensed for use in minors. The role of medication in children currently remains unclear and any contemplation of use should be referred to a specialist paediatrician.

9.22 Is there a role for bariatric surgery?

Bariatric, or obesity surgery (*see Chapter 8*), has been contemplated for children. If it has any role at all, it would be a treatment option of last resort and considered only in those children in whom medical weight management, delivered by a specialist centre, has failed to produce significant benefit. In addition, it could only be appropriate in children who are at imminent risk of serious comorbid disease and death. The author is unaware of any centres in the UK currently offering bariatric surgery to minors as a routine procedure but it is likely, as the numbers of obese children grow worldwide, that the possibility of such procedures becomes a reality.

9.23 Do residential courses work?

Residential weight management or activity courses (also called 'fat camps'; *see Q 6.28*) have been pioneered in the US and have found limited acceptance in Europe. One such camp in the UK – in Leeds – offers participating children a 6-week residential course. The children are encouraged, in a supportive and positive environment, to modify their dietary habits and activity levels, the aim being to develop sustainable changes that can be maintained long after return to normal family and school life. Results have been encouraging, with average total reductions being achieved in total body mass (7% decrease), BMI (7% decrease) and body fat (7% decrease) and increases in aerobic fitness averaging 21%.

9.24 What evidence exists of successful approaches in children?

The evidence for the effectiveness of weight-management programmes in children is sketchy and often disappointing. Many publications attempt to compare the efficacy of the different approaches but comparisons are difficult and therefore any conclusions need to be treated with caution. Clearly, more work needs to be done. Below are only a handful of examples.

SCHOOL-BASED PROGRAMMES

These encourage increased physical activity, either through structured educational initiatives or through teacher-led exercise schemes. They tend not to show significantly improved outcomes. Multifaceted programmes incorporating teacher-led, dietary and physical activity modification programmes, and alterations to the school curriculum and playground activities tend to be more successful. One such programme – Planet Health – aimed at children aged 11–13 years and conducted for 18 months, produced an overall reduction in obesity levels among girls and reduced TV watching in both boys and girls.

FAMILY-BASED PROGRAMMES

Results of family based studies vary considerably. Studies of programmes promoting healthy eating and physical activity seem to produce improvements in nutrition but not necessarily in weight. However, programmes that actively increase physical activity and dietary modification, and specifically target sedentary behaviour, might produce improved weight management. Epstein et al (1995) showed some benefit of dietary interventions and exercise at 6 months, compared with dietary education alone, but at 12 months the differences were not significant.

BEHAVIOUR MODIFICATION PROGRAMMES

Family-based programmes where the parents take the lead role for empowering dietary and activity level changes have been shown to help children to lose weight. In one study in the US – called Shapedown – significant weight decreases were achieved over a 15-month programme. Another study by Epstein et al (1987) encouraged improved parenting skills in obese children. At 12 months, significant weight improvements were observed but these were not maintained at 24 months.

PHARMACOLOGICAL INTERVENTIONS

Several small, short-term studies have found weight loss drugs to be of benefit but no guidance currently exists for the use of these drugs in weight management in childhood. The US National Institute of Child Health and Human Development is currently undertaking a randomly controlled trial in teenagers. Current opinion would suggest that the role of medication in children might be limited to adjunctive support in attaining weight maintenance and, in any case, limited to specialist paediatric weight-management clinics.

 PATIENT QUESTIONS

9.25 How can I tell if my child is overweight?

The standard measure of course is the Body Mass Index, but this can be difficult to calculate and you may not have access to the necessary centile charts. If you suspect your child is overweight your family doctor should be able to assess this for you. However, in my experience if parents suspect a problem they are usually right. Ask yourself (or your child) the following questions: Do they run around the playground with the other kids? Do they take part in school games? Do they get out of breath when running much earlier than their friends? Do they get teased by the other kids about their weight? Do the right size of clothes for their age fit easily? If the answers to these questions cause you concern, you will need to take some professional advice.

9.26 I don't want to medicalize the problem. What can I do to help my child myself?

First of all, don't panic. Don't allow your child to sense your worry. Take an apparently relaxed approach. Are they aware of the problem? Ask them the kind of questions given in the answer above. Your aim should be to assist them to become more active and to eat more healthily. To become more active, you may have to lead by example! Try walking more as a family, encourage outdoor play, limit car use, and make TV a time-limited exercise. Try and develop a healthier diet – for the whole family. Avoid sugary snacks, keep sweets as a one-a-week treat, try and encourage increased fruit and vegetable consumption, avoid fatty foods, and keep chips to a once-a-week event. Remember to be patient – think long term. Most importantly, don't isolate your child. Make them feel good about themselves, never guilty, and if in any doubt, get professional help.

The weight management clinic

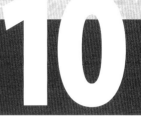

10

10.1 What are the benefits of weight loss?

The benefits of intentional weight loss can be very significant. In addition to the directly physiological changes, improvements in disease risk markers, there is also an improvement in comorbid disease control and, not to be forgotten, the very profound psychological benefits that can follow.

In 1997, Jung published estimates of the benefits of intentional weight loss. He estimated the effects of 10% body weight loss, that being an average of 10-kg weight loss in subjects averaging 100 kg in weight. The projected benefits are shown in *Table 10.1 (see also Box 3.1).*

> Jung's study also recognized that a 10% loss of bodyweight produced a >50% decrease in the risk of developing type 2 diabetes, a fall in fasting glucose levels of between 30 and 50%, and a 15% decrease in HbA$_1$c. Clinical experience shows that even a 5% bodyweight loss can produce quite profound benefits and many patients will express subjective improvements of decreased breathlessness, less weight-bearing joint pain, more energy and a more positive outlook.

To achieve these long-term health benefits, initial weight loss has to be maintained. In developing any weight-loss programme the emphasis must be on long-term weight management, and this has proven to be the greater challenge over early weight-loss success. The long-term prospects for those who are able to maintain their weight loss can be very significant. Hypertensive patients might be able to manage their hypertension and find they no longer require a prescription of antihypertensive agents. Type 1 diabetics might be able to reduce their insulin dosage levels, type 2 diabetics

TABLE 10.1 Benefits of a 10% loss in body weight	
Mortality	>20% fall in total mortality
	>30% fall in diabetes-related deaths
	>40% fall in obesity-related deaths
Blood pressure	Fall of 10 mmHg systolic and
	20 mmHg diastolic pressure
Diabetes	>50% decreased risk of developing diabetes
	30–50% fall in fasting glucose
	15% decrease in HbA$_1$c
Lipids	10% decrease in total cholesterol
	15% decrease in LDL
	30% decrease in triglycerides
	8% increase in HDL

might decrease and even remove their need for hypoglycaemic agents. Additionally, they are highly likely to delay the onset of cardiovascular disease and to improve their life expectancy.

However, many experts would emphasize that the improvements are best seen as a means of delaying disease and long-term monitoring of those at risk is essential. Recent research would suggest that those who are obese at the age of 40, despite long-term weight loss, do carry a decrease in life expectancy of approximately 3 years.

10.2 What constitutes an ideal weight-management clinic?

The ideal clinic should be able to:

- Deliver a weight-loss programme that is tailored to the individual.
- Offer regular and ongoing support.
- Embrace treatment modalities ranging from patient self-help groups and publications to commercial weight loss programmes.
- Offer lifestyle change support from specialist nurses, dieticians and physicians.
- Provide access to specialist dietetic advice.
- Offer specialist advice on increasing physical activity levels.
- Prescribe modern weight-loss pharmaceutical agents.
- Advise on the application of bariatric surgery techniques.

Such weight-loss programmes can be delivered in either primary or secondary care. The correct approach to individual patient management varies depending on the level of expertise and the facilities available.

An ideal clinic would be at a dedicated and specific time when obese patients would be able to make an appointment to see their clinician. Some patients, often for reasons of embarrassment, prefer not to attend surgery during normal routine clinic times because they think they would look out of place in the company of much leaner patients in the waiting room setting. However, this might not be practical and many clinics that are already delivering weight management services are 'rolling clinics' that obese patients are invited to attend during normal general medical clinic times.

10.3 What equipment is required?

It is essential that wide chairs, without restrictive arms, are available in the consulting room. Basic clinical measurements will include height, weight and blood pressure. It is essential that regularly calibrated scales, to a minimum of 200 kg, are available. Sphygmomanometers with a large-sized cuff are essential for accurate blood pressure measurements in the obese. Other equipment should include a waist tape, often specially designed for the purpose, and – ideally – equipment to measure body fat mass. Supportive literature to give to the patient is always welcome.

10.4 How do you raise the issue with the patient?

Many health professionals express concern about how a patient will react if the issue of overweight and obesity is raised. They fear that it could damage the doctor–patient relationship. This sensitivity on the part of health professionals reflects the difficulties to be found in discussing obesity not just within a clinic setting but also in society in general.

In the author's experience the majority of patients understand the reason for raising the subject, do not take offence and are often only too pleased that the doctor or nurse has expressed an interest and understanding of the significance obesity has on their potential disease development.

In raising the issue of obesity it is important that the clinician exercises good communication skills, finds the right language to use in that particular context, avoids the use of medical jargon and puts the effects of obesity in context with the rest of the patient's medical history. For example, a patient is unlikely to embrace the concept of weight loss as a means of dealing with their type 2 diabetes if the role of medication (which would perhaps be their first expectation) is not discussed and put into context. The clinician needs to address the patient's concern, discuss how much support is to be offered and to establish an agreed approach towards weight loss.

10.5 What goals should be set?

It is absolutely essential that, from the outset, the patient and the clinician share the realistic expectations of what weight loss might be achieved. One specialist clinic asked female patients how much weight they expected to lose. The average response was 37% of their total body weight. They said they would consider a 25% bodyweight loss as satisfactory, would be reluctant to accept 17% and would be disappointed with only 10%. It is therefore quite common that at initial presentation the first appointment turns into disappointment, as the patient is helped to recognize more realistic goals. Of course, it is possible for patients to lose much more than 10% body weight, even as much as 40–50%, but this is uncommon and the vast majority of patients should reasonably expect to be able to lose and maintain 10% of their body weight.

The medical benefits of this 10% weight loss should be emphasized to the patient (and the clinician!) and should help promote acceptance. The concept of attempting to return the patients to their 'ideal weight' is outdated and should be unceremoniously dumped. The use of 'ideal weight' as a target is highly likely to lead to unrealistic and unachievable weight loss goals and ultimate failure. It is important that, from the outset, the initial aim of the weight management programme should be stressed to be modest weight loss followed by weight maintenance.

For the majority of obese adults a weight loss goal of 10% over a period of 3–6 months is achievable. This could be achieved by losing 0.5–1 kg per week on average. This would lead, on average, to weight loss of anywhere between 5 and 20 kg and would require a kcal deficit of 500–600 kcal to be achieved daily.

Many patients will express disappointment at this projected rate of weight loss, describing it as 'too slow'. This needs to be addressed at the outset, perhaps by encouraging them to consider that as weight *gain* has occurred over a prolonged period, weight *loss* should also be a gradual process. Even at a rate of weight loss of 1–2 lb per week, weight reduction will be much more rapid than the original gain. Additionally, it is recognized that those who lose weight rapidly are more likely to regain afterwards. In arriving at agreed weight loss goals with the patient, the following measures of progress should also be discussed:

- appropriate weight loss
- avoiding subsequent weight regain
- management of other risk factors
- improvements in mental and emotional well-being.

10.6 What is 'readiness to change'?

'Readiness to change' is described by psychologists as the level of preparedness of an individual to make significant lifestyle alterations to promote a sustained change in the energy balance equation to achieve long-term weight loss. Readiness to change is so important that if an individual is thought to be unprepared to change, perhaps because of current social circumstances, employment or financial hardship, such as redundancy or buying a home, weight loss might not be a sufficiently high priority to commit to the challenging behavioural change that would be required. In these circumstances, it would be reasonable to encourage the individual to commit his or her energies to the greater priorities and to return for weight-management advice when he or she feels able to embrace the changes required.

Readiness to change can be assessed in a variety of ways. Sophisticated psychological models are used in some specialist centres but, despite what appears to be 'readiness', an individual's circumstances might change within a very short space of time. There is therefore no sufficiently accurate method to predict those who are likely to succeed.

Within a primary care setting, the doctor or nurse is in prime position to have a good knowledge of a patient's past medical history, social situation and personality profile. It is therefore perhaps more prudent to make a decision on the patient's readiness dependent upon your discussions plus background knowledge.

10.7 What motivates change?

Human nature is such that if someone tells you what to do there is a high chance that you will do the opposite! Patients need to be able to see for themselves the importance of lifestyle change, and the benefits it could bestow. It is important that clinicians do not overly influence patients, but rather seek to facilitate patients in expressing *their* reasons for change, and *their* motivation for doing so.

It is important to establish with the patient that there are significant changes that they are able to make that will produce effective results. It is wrong to expect patients to immediately embrace any suggestions. Ambivalence towards change is normal and a natural part of the behaviour-changing process. Decision making involves patients weighing up the pros and cons for themselves, and this can take time. It is highly likely, however, that the prospects of success are directly proportional to the enthusiasm of not just the patients but also their clinician.

10.8 How do you assess readiness to change?

It is essential to establish good rapport, to increase your understanding of the reasons for the patient presenting, perhaps to become familiar with previous dieting and attempts at weight loss, and to develop an understanding of the difficulties and barriers the patient faces in attempting any further weight management.

Discussing previous weight management attempts can highlight a patient's beliefs and understanding about his or her weight and allow the clinician to address any negative thoughts and concerns. It provides an opportunity to discuss patient expectations and agree the way forward.

10.9 Who should be offered weight management?

In selecting which patients are to be offered weight management, it is helpful to consider what is to be achieved. Do you intend to offer weight management to every patient with a BMI >30? Or perhaps your priority is patients with a BMI >27 but with the presence of comorbid disease?

Many patients self-present and ask for help with weight management but many more do not and it will be up to the clinician to raise the issue of weight management when they present with their related, or even unrelated, disease. In a primary care setting almost 50% of patients with hypertension will be obese, 33% of those with ischaemic heart disease patients will be obese and 85% of type 2 diabetics are likely to be overweight.

For a clinician considering setting up a new obesity clinic, the thought of dealing with the approximately 20% of the adult population who are clinically obese is daunting. However, in the author's experience, at any one time less than half of this 20% is concerned enough to accept weight management advice and of these, perhaps half again will choose to attempt weight loss through their own means, perhaps using commercial agencies. The clinician can therefore be selective when prioritizing patients, particularly if it is thought that delivering weight management to all appropriate patients would be too daunting a task to even start.

But what is to be your priority? Obesity treatment *per se*? Or perhaps prevention and improved management of comorbid disease by medically assisted weight reduction? Individual clinicians should assess their own patient population needs and decide their own priorities.

10.10 What clinical investigations are required?

Clinical investigation is required to isolate any pre-existing medical pathology such as type 2 diabetes. It serves as a baseline for future reference to monitor a progressive decrease in comorbid disease risk markers, and also to establish the current level of control of pre-existing comorbid diseases such as hypertension and dyslipaedemia. Clinical investigations are also useful for reassuring patients that there is no reason why they should not be able to lose weight. The most common reasons patients give for not being able to lose weight are: 'I've got an underactive thyroid', 'I'm just big boned', 'It's in my genes' and 'I've always been this way'.

> Physical investigation should include height, weight and BMI. Additionally, waist circumference, blood pressure and urinalysis are essential; measurement of body fat mass is desirable.
> Biochemical investigation should include thyroid function tests, liver function, fasting glucose and fasting lipids and, when indicated (for example when PCOS is suspected), sex hormones analysis.
> Chest X-ray, ECG, a glucose tolerance test and 24-hour urinary cortisol are not usually indicated but might become essential to further investigate concerns raised during history taking or physical examination.

10.11 What can patients do to help themselves?

By presenting to your weight-management clinic and asking for help, patients have already made the first positive statement that they are taking weight management seriously. After establishing what previous attempts at weight loss have been made, you might find that the patient is very informed about the energy balance equation and the multitude of approaches towards weight loss. However, your unique contribution will be a medicalization of the problem, added professional support for long-term success and concomitant management of any comorbid disease.

It is helpful to give the patient supportive literature, in the form of either a book or leaflets, and perhaps access to supportive and reliable websites.

Asking patients to prepare a food diary is an excellent tool in further assessing the level of motivation and kick starting their understanding of their own dietary habits and need for change. Ask patients to commit to writing down everything that they eat or drink, in detail for 1 week, and to return to you with a completed food diary. In the process of doing this, several changes occur:

1. Patients very quickly become aware of trends in their own eating habits. For example, patients might know they were having a biscuit with every cup of tea but think that one biscuit is not important. Keeping a food diary can foster a realization of the cumulative effect these biscuits – five cups of tea a day for seven days a week soon amounts to a significant number of unnecessary calories!
2. Second, the patient is highly likely to have started to implement some change before returning to see you.
3. Third, a diary is a very valuable tool when you are working with the patient to establish some simple changes that might produce profound changes in dietary calorific intake.

Patients who fail to complete a food diary were probably not sufficiently motivated or ready for change at the current time.

10.12 What comes next?

The patient has presented to you, or you have initiated the discussion and it has been agreed that weight loss would be highly advantageous either to prevent comorbid disease development or improve control of existing comorbid disease. You have assessed the patient's readiness to change, level of motivation and past history of weight-loss attempts. You will have developed an understanding of the patient's social and medical history, established the existence (or level of control) of comorbid disease and have presented the patient with a few obstacles to overcome to demonstrate his or her seriousness and desire for long-term weight loss.

For many patients, the amount of support already offered and the expression of serious intent by the clinician at this early stage will have a profound effect on their levels of motivation and determination to success in the long term. The impact of the degree of support offered by the clinician should never be underestimated. You will have set reasonable goals and expectations for short-term weight loss and subsequent weight maintenance, and will hopefully have agreed with the patient the appropriate way forward. In an ideal world, 2-weekly appointments would be offered, in the real world perhaps monthly is more acceptable. Alternating appointments between a doctor and nurse might be considered, together with referral for special dietetic or physical activity advice. It is thereafter appropriate to move forward towards making changes to dietary intake and physical activity levels to promote a negative change in energy balance equation, to promote weight loss. The patient is ready to start.

The role of primary care

11

11.1 How does obesity impact on primary care?

Obesity has major financial implications for primary care. Obese patients are likely to consult their family doctor at least 30% more often than lean adults. They also account for approximately 30% greater prescribing costs. Many obese patients with type 2 diabetes or cardiovascular disease are treated with a multitude of medications to control their blood pressure, dyslipidaemia, hyperglycaemia and ischaemic heart disease. Achieving recommended blood pressure levels in diabetics will usually require one-third to be on one medication, two-thirds to be on two medications and one-third to be on three. Virtually all type 2 diabetics would be prescribed a statin to improve lipid profile. The combination of obesity, dyslipidaemia, hypertension and impaired glucose tolerance, often combined in the 'metabolic syndrome' (*see Q 3.14*) affects around 25% of adults in the US and similar numbers in the UK. Primary care is already heavily involved in treating chronic obesity induced disease and enduring the costs of doing so.

11.2 What is the role of primary care in the management of obesity?

Primary care should have the central role in the medical management of obesity (*see Q 8.15*). It is the first port of call for patients who consult about their weight, about a comorbidity of their weight or about totally unrelated matters. In the first two categories it is the GP's role to actively assess and help patients manage their weight, and in the last to opportunistically flag up overweight as a problem, if it is appropriate and practical to do so.

Many obese patients already attend regular surgery clinics, for example diabetic or heart disease clinics, so weight management is either already taking place or can quite conveniently be undertaken. In such patients, weight management is an essential element of overall treatment, as reducing weight helps control all risk markers; cholesterol, blood pressure, blood glucose, and so on. Alternatively, a practice audit might unearth patients with raised BMI who merit treatment.

Many practices look after their obese patients in a dedicated weight-management clinic. This might be convenient in larger practices but it is not essential for good individual management of any one patient. Weight management should, in any event, be shared by as many members of the primary care team as possible, who should all be well-versed in the importance of the condition and the different facets of its treatment.

In most areas of the UK there is limited or no access to specialist hospital obesity clinics, which places obesity management even more emphatically on the GPs plate, but the primary care team should, in any case, be familiar with the use of second-line measures such as drug therapy. Antiobesity pharmacotherapy is safe and effective and, like basic drug management of any chronic disease, can be used in day-to-day general practice without reliance on consultant referrals.

11.3 Why should GPs treat obesity?

It is essential that obesity is treated actively in primary care. The benefits of even a moderate degree of weight loss are extremely significant and act as a good illustration that obesity is closely associated with a wide range of clinical conditions.

11.4 What guidelines are available for obesity management?

The National Obesity Forum guidelines are the most applicable to primary care management of obesity, as they are written by primary care professionals and are intended to be of practical use in a busy general practice to assist decision making. They are evidence based and concise. There are currently three sets of NOF guidelines:

- National Obesity Forum guidelines on management of adult obesity and overweight in primary care
- An approach to weight management in children and adolescents (2–18 years) in primary care, formulated in partnership with the Royal College of Paediatrics and Child Health
- National Obesity Forum pharmacotherapy guidelines for obesity management in adults

These are available via the NOF or from its website (http://www.nationalobesityforum.org.uk) and are reproduced in the Appendix.

11.5 What are the other important guidelines?

The Scottish Intercollegiate Guidelines Network (SIGN) has produced guidelines for the management of obesity in both adults and children. These are extremely thorough and comprehensive as a reference, although secondary care based.

In 2003, the Royal College of Physicians produced influential guidelines entitled *Antiobesity drugs guidance on appropriate prescribing and management*, which (like the SIGN guidelines) are produced by, and aimed at, secondary care professionals.

NICE has produced guidelines for the use of antiobesity pharmacotherapy for orlistat and sibutramine and for the use of bariatric surgery. Currently, NICE is collecting evidence for an appraisal of the overall management of obesity.

National Service Frameworks (NSFs) for coronary heart disease and diabetes have been produced in the UK and highlight the importance of obesity management as part of treatment of the respective conditions.

There are various important sources of guidance in the US, including the National Institutes of Health (NHLBI) and the National Cholesterol Education Program (NCEP), which defined the metabolic syndrome. The Surgeon General's *Call to action to prevent and decrease overweight and obesity* is available at http://www.surgeongeneral.gov. Internationally, the WHO has issued many important documents relating to obesity, diet, health and nutrition, most notably *Obesity: preventing and managing the global epidemic* and *Diet, nutrition and the prevention of chronic diseases: report of a joint WHO/FAO expert consultation*.

In the UK, the government initiated debate on the subject of obesity when it published *The health of the nation*. More recently, in 2001, the National Audit Office produced a report identifying the problems associated with obesity. This report includes the economic costs, sets out examples of good practice and suggest policies for the future. It is available at http://www.nao.gov.uk/pn/00-01/0001220.htm. In 2002 the All-Party Parliamentary Group on Obesity was formed and in 2003 the government launched a Health Select Committee studying obesity in the UK.

Other important sources of information include leaflets such as the *Balance of good health*, which spells out good diet and nutrition, with information on the amount of fruit, vitamins and minerals. This, or similar guidelines, should be readily available to hand out to patients along with information about physical activity, including local sources. US dietary guidelines can be found at http://www.health.gov/dietaryguidelines.

The future

12.1 What advances are likely in obesity management?

The future of obesity management depends primarily on four factors:

1. The quality of care offered by the medical profession, especially primary care.
2. The commercial 'slimming industry'.
3. The changes made to the current 'toxic' environment.
4. Advances within the pharmaceutical industry.

What changes are likely to occur in the medical management of obesity?

Statistics make it very clear that medical management of obesity has not yet succeeded in reversing the current epidemic; there is no sign of a slowing down in the increasing prevalence of the condition. This might be partly because many patients – notoriously young and middle aged men – do not present to us with weight problems in the first place, and partly because time constraints and lack of resources in general practice make it impossible for us to devote enough attention to the condition as we would like.

Obesity is not always well managed by the medical or nursing professions. Only 20% of obese patients ever receive treatment and, when they do, it is often from a doctor who has a negative attitude towards obesity, lacks confidence, is dissatisfied with treating obesity because of its 90% 'failure' rate and is unaware of up-to-date treatment strategies (Haslam 2000). With increasing recognition of the metabolic syndrome and the central role of obesity in a wide variety of conditions and comorbidities, obesity will inevitably be considered a greater priority in day-to-day practice, in GP contracts and in primary care guidelines.

For the epidemic of obesity to be tackled successfully, primary care professionals not only need to be well informed about the condition and motivated to treat it, but also need to have sufficient time and resources to devote sufficient attention to its management.

12.2 What is happening in the world of the commercial slimming industry?

The multibillion pound world of private and commercial slimming products is beyond the scope of this book. It is also impossible to predict the effect that market forces will have on the industry in the years to come, when obesity will be even more widespread than it is today. However, it seems likely that the growing number of safe and effective entities, be they slimming groups, books, clinics, telephone helplines or internet sites, will need to collaborate with each other, and with the medical profession, to provide for the many millions of potential customers. In fact, commercial weight-loss organizations are increasingly seeking collaborative involvement with the medical professions, sharing expertise and giving a greater emphasis to medical, rather than cosmetic, weight loss.

12.3 Will the current 'toxic' environment ever change?

The obesogenic environment in which we currently live is the major cause of the obesity epidemic, and for any advances to be made in the fight against the condition it is essential that changes occur. At the time of writing, major players in the food industry and in the UK government are beginning to make changes in policies (*see* Q 2.22), which suggests that there is a glimmer of hope for the future.

12.4 What pharmaceutical developments are imminent?

It is difficult to assess the current state of pharmaceutical developments in the fight against obesity, as many drugs that appear to be on the verge of being the next great breakthrough fall by the wayside, whereas others appear from nowhere to gain approval on the 'fast track'. More than 100 molecules are currently undergoing detailed research.

Some examples of possible areas in research or development are outlined in *Box 12.1*.

12.5 What is likely to be the next available antiobesity drug?

Rimonabant (or Acomplia) is in a new class of drug entitled selective CB1 blocker, which is in the final stages of studies for treatment of both obesity and smoking. It blocks the CB1 receptors in the endocannabinoid (EC) system, which has a role in regulation of body weight and lipid metabolism. The receptors are found both in the brain and peripherally, such as in adipose tissue. Increased activity of the system is associated with excessive food intake, and fat accumulation as well as with smoking. Rimonabant inhibits the increased activity of the system, causing weight loss and substantial metabolic benefits. The Rimonabant in Obesity (RIO) study followed patients for one year taking 20 mg rimonabant compared with placebo, and demonstrated a loss of 8.6 kg, compared with 2.3 kg on placebo. Almost 75% of patients lost at least 5% of their body weight (compared to placebo; 27.6%) and 44.3% lost at least 10% (placebo; 10.3%).

The metabolic benefits are summarized below:

- 9.1 cm reduction in waist circumference
- Increase of 23% in HDL
- Reduction of 15% in LDL
- Increase in size of LDL particles, therefore reduced cardiovascular risk
- CRP reduced by 27% compared to 11% in placebo group
- Improved insulin sensitivity.
- The number of patients diagnosed with metabolic syndrome at baseline was halved after treatment

It seems likely that rimonabant will become a useful addition to the pharmacotherapy arsenal, and may have a particular role to play in avoiding weight gain in those people quitting smoking.

12.6 What is lipodystrophy?

Lipodystrophy is a condition in which adipose tissue is laid down abnormally – in excess quantities in some parts of the body, for example the trunk and neck, and in reduced amounts in the extremities. Some researchers believe that study of the aetiology of the various forms of lipodystrophy, coupled with their associated metabolic abnormalities, might unlock many of the mysteries of obesity and help find a solution.

Lipodystrophy can be inherited or acquired, and can vary from being a minor cosmetic problem to a catastrophic metabolic disorder. The inherited forms of lipodystrophy are caused by gene defects and include congenital generalized lipodystrophy and familial partial lipodystrophy. The most notable of the acquired forms is highly active antiretroviral therapy (HAART)-induced lipodystrophy, which is a side-effect of HIV treatment. But other forms, such as acquired generalized lipodystrophy and acquired parital lipodystrophy might be autoimmune disorders; their aetiologies are uncertain. The conditions have in common exaggerated, extreme and accelerated manifestations of insulin resistance and its complications, which include raised blood levels of insulin, glucose, cholesterol and triglycerides, and result in severe risk of diabetes, coronary heart disease stroke, etc.

BOX 12.1 Current areas of research and development

- Glucose tolerance factor: a chromium-based substance required for normal glucose tolerance. This has stimulated interest in chromium supplementation, e.g. brewer's yeast
- US research has suggested that obesity is a hypothalamic disorder: hypothalamic long-chain fatty acids decrease food intake and reduce glucose production in the liver
- Bupropion (Zyban®) is currently used for smoking cessation but is undergoing trials for effects on weight loss
- Axokine is a drug in stage II trials, it might be useful for inducing weight loss in type 2 diabetics
- Diazoxide is thought to induce weight loss in women with PCOS
- Naltrexone is currently used for drug and alcohol dependency. It might have an effect on obesity, as might the antidepressant sertraline
- The anticonvulsant topiramide was thought to induce weight loss but trials have been discontinued. Another antiseizure drug –

zonisamide – has been shown to induce weight loss compared to placebo
- More than two-dozen newly recognized gut hormones have been isolated. These control appetite and energy metabolism and might represent promising pathways for developing new treatments for obesity and type 2 diabetes
- Orexin is a newly discovered compound that appears to be generated when blood sugar levels drop. It acts as a trigger to eating. The name is derived from the Greek orexis, meaning 'appetite'
- Galanin is a neuropeptide that is thought to be part of the regulatory system in the control of body weight
- Leptin is still being studied for its effect on weight loss. It is thought it might be useful in combination with VLCDs to minimize the effect of hunger
- Amylin is a hormone that is secreted alongside insulin. It is involved with glucose regulation. Its effect on weight are being evaluated
- Hundreds of chromosomes and genes are still being assessed for their role in the aetiology of obesity and it seems likely that multiple genetic variations are responsible for a tendency to obesity in an individual
- The ancient alternative therapy bitter melon has hypoglycaemic properties and a possible role in weight management
- The effect of growth hormone (GH) on obesity is being studied. GH levels are known to be low in obesity and injecting a daily dose of the hormone might prevent accumulation of fat
- The hormone PYY, which is produced by the intestine in response to eating and tells the brain when enough has been eaten, is considered to be an important discovery with potential for drug development
- Another gut peptide, cholecystokinin, reduces gastric emptying (and therefore appetite), as does glucagon-like peptide 1
- Dopamine agonists such as cabergoline and bromocriptine have been noted to cause weight loss and are under investigation as potential weight-loss drugs. Various B_3 adrenergic receptor agonists are under development. It is hoped that these will improve insulin sensitivity
- Extracts of South African cacti (known as P57) containing steroidal glycosides have appetite-suppressant characteristics and are advancing through trial stages

Professional groups

THE NATIONAL OBESITY FORUM (NOF)

The National Obesity Forum was established in May 2000 to raise awareness of the growing impact of obesity and overweight on patients and professionals in the UK. Membership is open to all healthcare professionals and is free. The NOF aims to increase the availability of best practice in weight management across the medical professions by using all available resources in the media – politically, educationally and professionally – to enable practitioners to treat overweight patients confidently and well (see NOF guidelines in Appendix, and also at the website address listed below). Regular newsletters and an active website ensure the professional membership is kept in touch with recent developments. The aims and objectives of the National Obesity Forum include:

- To create recognition of obesity as a serious medical problem.
- To provide education and training on weight management.
- To produce and update guidelines for weight management within primary care.
- To campaign politically and in the media for better understanding and support for obese patients and those providing them with medical care.
- To provide a network for health professionals and an obesity management support and information resource.
- To convince government and healthcare workers to give obesity a high priority nationally and locally.
- To support the annual 'Excellence in weight management best practice award'.

The NOF supports and provides professional advice to the All-Party Parliamentary Group on Obesity and provides guidance to NICE, the HDA and the Health Select Committee.

WEB ADDRESS
http://www.nationalobesityforum.org.uk

THE ASSOCIATION FOR THE STUDY OF OBESITY (ASO)

The Association for the Study of Obesity (ASO) was founded in 1967 and was the UK's first professional organization dedicated to the understanding and treatment of obesity. The ASO has three key objectives:

1. To promote research into the causes, prevention and treatment of obesity. This includes the presentation of annual awards to researchers in the field for individual contributions and best practice.
2. To encourage action to reduce the prevalence of obesity and to enhance treatment.
3. To facilitate contact between health professionals and organizations interested in any aspect of obesity and bodyweight regulation.

The ASO was the founding body of the highly respected *International Journal of Obesity* and is affiliated to the European and International Associations for the Study of Obesity. Membership of the ASO is open to scientists, medical and health professionals working within the field of obesity. Members receive free registration at key ASO meetings, ASO newsletters, affiliation to International Association for the Study of Obesity (IASO) and European Association for the Study of Obesity (EASO).

WEB ADDRESS

http://www.aso.org.uk

DIETITIANS IN OBESITY MANAGEMENT UK (DOM)

A specialist group, providing expertise in clinical, public health approaches to weight management and professional training for dietitians and other interested health professionals. Its aim is to aid the development of best practice in dietetic care of the obese, within the context of integrated care, to improve prevention and management and thereby reduce the impact of obesity in the UK. Membership is open to all state registered dietitians.

WEB ADDRESS

http://www.bda.uk.com/membership/interestgroup

THE INTERNATIONAL OBESITY TASK FORCE (IOTF)

The IOTF was founded in response to a growing recognition of the need to promote obesity as a serious health risk with worldwide implications. Part of the International Association for the Study of Obesity, the IOTF works with the WHO and obesity specialists throughout the world to inform the medical and political world of the growing health crisis caused by obesity. Its focus is on prevention, treatment, cost consequences and childhood obesity. The IOTF has been instrumental in persuading governments to change their policies towards obesity and it continues to produce groundbreaking reports used by health professionals the world over to influence practice and prevention.

WEB ADDRESS

http://www.iotf.org

THE SPECIALIST CERTIFICATION OF OBESITY PROFESSIONALS IN EUROPE (SCOPE)

SCOPE is an IOTF–European Association for the Study of Obesity initiative designed to improve the treatment of the obese patient in Europe. The goals of SCOPE are:

1. To identify experts in the management of obesity and create a European registry of SCOPE fellows.
2. To enhance the quality of obesity education in Europe by providing summer schools and online courses.
3. To expand this training programme to a wider range of health professionals.
4. To improve treatment of the obese and overweight patient.

Launched at the European Congress on Obesity in Helsinki in 2003, SCOPE aims to provide training courses for GPs and specialist physicians with a view to qualification for either fellowship or membership. Interactive educational website courses are also planned.

WEB ADDRESS

http://www.iotf.org and follow links to SCOPE.

NATIONAL INSTITUTE FOR CLINICAL EXCELLENCE (NICE)

Although it is part of the NHS, NICE is an independent organization responsible for providing national guidance on treatments and care in England and Wales. Its guidance is for healthcare professionals, patients and carers, and is designed to enable decisions about treatment and healthcare. NICE guidance and recommendations are prepared by independent groups that include professionals working in the NHS and people who are familiar with the issues affecting patients and carers. As part of its review process, NICE has reviewed the evidence for weight-management therapies, with particular reference to the use of medication, orlistat and sibutramine, and bariatric surgery. Full details can be found on their website. Clinical guidelines for weight management are planned.

WEB ADDRESS

http://www.nice.org.uk

SCOTTISH INTERCOLLEGIATE GUIDELINES NETWORK (SIGN)

SIGN was formed in 1993. The objective of SIGN is to improve the quality of healthcare for patients in Scotland by reducing variation in practice and outcome through the development and dissemination of national clinical guidelines containing recommendations for effective practice based on current evidence. The membership of SIGN includes all the medical specialties, nursing, pharmacy, dentistry, professions allied to medicine, patients, health service managers, social services and researchers, and is supported by the Royal College of Physicians of Edinburgh. The SIGN guideline development programme is funded by the Clinical Resource and Audit Group (CRAG) of the Scottish Executive Health Department.

SIGN has developed guidelines for weight management in children and adult obesity. These evidence-based guidelines are derived from a systematic review of the scientific evidence and, they say, are therefore less susceptible to bias in their conclusions and recommendations. Published in 1996, the SIGN guidelines on obesity are thought to be the most widely read weight-management guidelines in the world.

WEB ADDRESS

http://www.sign.ac.uk

ROYAL COLLEGE OF PAEDIATRICS AND CHILD HEALTH

WEB ADDRESS

http://www.rcpch.ac.uk

ROYAL COLLEGE OF PHYSICIANS

WEB ADDRESS

http://www.rcplondon.ac.uk

Patient support and information

WEIGHT CONCERN

A charitable group, Weight Concern was founded in 1997 by Professor Jane Wardle and Lorna Rapoport of the Clinical Psychology Unit at the University College Hospital, London. Recognizing the need for an organization for overweight people, they attracted a team of like-minded health professionals and overweight people. Weight Concern aims to address the physical and psychological problems of the overweight, and to guide development of more effective programmes of prevention and treatment. Other aims include:

■ the advancement of public knowledge about the causes, consequences and treatments of weight problems
■ the provision of advocacy and advice for overweight people
■ the provision of education and training for health professionals in the care of overweight patients.

WEB ADDRESS

http://www.weightconcern.com

TOAST

The Obesity Awareness and Solutions Trust – TOAST – was founded in 1998 and is a national UK charity dedicated to encouraging a better understanding of obesity, its causes and the practical solutions that are (or should be) available. TOAST works predominantly in the public sector but is also involved in promoting better professional and political understanding. It seeks to encourage informed debate and research into obesity, and to stimulate action for its prevention and treatment. TOAST was the first charity in the UK to use action groups to inform, educate and listen to people with obesity. TOAST was formed to be a focus for a comprehensive strategy for the prevention and management of obesity in the UK, uniting the people who know with the people who need to know.

WEB ADDRESS

http://www.toast-uk.org.uk

THE CHILD GROWTH FOUNDATION (CGF)

The CGF is a charity dedicated to the support and relief of all persons (either children or adults) suffering from growth disorders and their families in any manner. It aims to promote and fund research into the causes and cure of disorders of growth in children within the area of benefit and to publish the results of such research to educate the public, in general, and workers in the medical profession, in particular, in the problems and difficulties encountered by those with growth disorders. The CGF has been a very active supporter of the importance of early detection and treatment of childhood obesity.

WEB ADDRESS

http://www.caritasdata.co.uk

THE EATING DISORDERS ASSOCIATION (EDA)

The EDA aims to be the leading organization providing information, help and support across the UK for people whose lives are affected by eating disorders. Their aim is to positively influence public understanding and policy. The key aims of the EDA are to:

■ Increase knowledge, awareness and understanding of eating disorders and EDA.
■ Provide information, help and support to all those affected by these illnesses.
■ Campaign for continually improved standards and availability of treatment and care for people with eating disorders.

Recognizing the clinical cross-over between obesity and eating disorders, EDA is a crucial voice in the obesity debate.

WEB ADDRESS

http://edauk.com

THE MEN'S HEALTH FORUM

The Men's Health Forum was founded in 1994 and gained charitable status in 2001. It is an independent body that works with a wide range of individuals and organizations to promote the issue of men's health. Its active membership aims to develop health services that will meet men's needs and enable men to change their risk-taking behaviour. The Men's Health Forum works to improve the health of men and men's health services through research and policy development, professional training, providing information services and stimulating professional and public debate. The Forum also works to further discussions with MPs and government, develop innovative and imaginative projects and collaboration with the widest possible range of interested organizations and individuals.

The Forum is also involved in organising national Men's Health Week each June, publishing the *Men's Health Journal*, providing a male health website aimed at health professionals, and holding an annual conference. It maintains a database of men's health projects throughout the UK and supports the work of the All-Party Parliamentary Group on Men's Health. Other aims of the Forum include:

- Running health-promotion and public education campaigns on a variety of issues, including erectile dysfunction and prostate disease.
- Providing the most comprehensive consumer health website dedicated to male health (malehealth.co.uk).
- Developing policy on preventing young male suicides and delivering training on suicide prevention to health professionals.
- Tackling gender inequalities through the Gender and Health Partnership.
- Playing an active role in the European Men's Health Forum.
- Working closely with the International Society for Men's Health.

WEB ADDRESS

http://www.menshealthforum.org.uk

OVEREATERS ANONYMOUS

Binge eating disorders are very prevalent among obese patients. Overeaters Anonymous is an international group offering a programme of recovery from compulsive overeating meetings. It provides what it describes as 'a fellowship of experience, strength and hope where members respect one another's anonymity'. Overeaters Anonymous does not charge fees but is self-supporting through member contributions.

Overeaters Anonymous focuses on more than just weight loss, obesity or diets; it aims to address physical, emotional and spiritual well-being. It is not a religious organization and does not promote any particular diet. To address weight loss, Overeaters Anonymous encourages members to develop a weight-management plan with a healthcare professional and a 'sponsor'. Patients who are seeking help with compulsive eating can find the support offered by Overeaters Anonymous to be beneficial.

WEB ADDRESS
http://www.oa.org

DIABETES UK

Diabetes UK is the leading charity working for people with diabetes, funding research and campaigns to help people to live with the condition. Its stated aim is to improve the lives of people with diabetes and to work towards a future without diabetes.

Diabetes UK's forerunner, the Diabetic Association, was set up in 1934 by novelist HG Wells and Dr RD Lawrence – both of whom had diabetes. The radical charity they founded aimed to ensure that everyone in the UK could gain access to insulin, whatever their financial situation. In addition, the Diabetic Association (which became the British Diabetic Association in 1954) challenged accepted ideas of how people should be treated. It campaigned for the foundation of the National Health Service and believed that people with diabetes should take an active role in managing their condition; in effect, promoting a patient-centred approach. In 1939, the Diabetic Association set up the first diabetes voluntary self-support group. This has now grown to a network of more than 400 local voluntary groups, which provide support and information to people with diabetes across the UK. The British Diabetic Association was renamed as Diabetes UK in 2000. Its aims include:

- improving the lives of those with diabetes
- ending discrimination and ignorance
- providing the best source of information on diabetes.

Membership is open to health care professionals and members of the public.

WEB ADDRESS
http://diabetes.org.uk

FOUNDATIONS

Foundations is the name of a new charity whose aim is to empower people to build a positive self-image and a healthy body.

Recognizing that eating disorders, obesity and lack of self-esteem are growing problems among teenagers and young adults, Foundations has had requests to provide preventive programmes for schools and adolescents to help them discuss issues about body image, nutrition and exercise. The objectives of Foundations are to:

- Empower people to make choices about eating and exercise from a standpoint of balanced information and self-awareness.
- Prevent eating problems from developing.
- Raise public awareness and campaign on public policy issues relating to health, eating problems and body image.
- Provide information relating to eating, exercise and body image.
- Provide training for all professionals and helpers working with eating problems, exercise and body image.
- Provide therapeutic help through counselling, groups and workshops.
- Raise public awareness of the complex issues relating to eating problems, exercise and body image.
- Understand and meet the needs of all groups and respect diversity in culture, age and gender.
- Include the many people who do not have an eating disorder but have a negative view of themselves or are caught in negative/unhealthy cycles.
- Establish research programmes relating to the complex issues of eating problems and body image.

WEB ADDRESS

http://www.eatingproblems.org

SUSTAIN

Sustain – the alliance for better food and farming – is a charitable group that 'advocates food and agriculture policies and practices that enhance the health and welfare of people and animals, improve the working and living environment, enrich society and culture and promote equity'. It represents over 100 national public interest organizations working at international, national, regional and local levels. In relation to obesity, Sustain has been at the forefront in the campaign to limit the advertising of obesogenic foods to children.

In collaboration with its membership, Sustain aims to facilitate the exchange of information to develop networks of members and allied organizations to devise and implement policies on particular issues of common concern. It has an extensive range of publications covering current and past areas of work.

Membership is open to national organizations that do not distribute profits to private shareholders and that therefore operate in the public interest. The organizations must be wholly or partly interested in food or farming issues and support the general aims and work of the alliance.

WEB ADDRESS

http://www.sustainweb.org

APPENDIX
Guidelines for managing obesity

National Obesity Forum guidelines on management of adult obesity and overweight in primary care*

Obesity and overweight can be managed in Primary Care by a motivated well-informed multi-disciplinary team. The aim of treatment is to achieve and maintain weight loss by promoting sustainable changes in lifestyle.

PATIENT SELECTION

Most patients attending diabetic or cardiovascular clinics will automatically be candidates for weight management. Other patients may be picked up by practice audit, opportunistic screening or self-referral. Posters and leaflets should be available in the surgery and community for the education of patients.

TREATMENT GROUPS

Treatment or advice should be offered to:

- Patients with BMI >30.
- Patients with BMI >28 with co-morbidities, e.g. COAD, coronary heart disease and diabetes.
- Patients with any degree of overweight coinciding with diabetes, other severe risk factors or serious disease.
- Patients who self-refer, where appropriate.
- Parents of families with more than one obese or overweight member may need special consideration and more intensive support.
- Prevention advice should be offered to high risk individuals, e.g. those with a family history of obesity, smokers, people with learning disabilities, low income groups.

HISTORY

Including personal medical history, family history, social history, past history of dieting, readiness to change, barriers to change and current diet and levels of activity.

INVESTIGATIONS

- To isolate any medical pathology.
- To act as a baseline for future measurements.

*These guidelines (and others, including those on managing childhood obesity) can be found in full on the NOF website, www.nationalobesityforum.org.uk

- To exclude any secondary conditions or comorbidities.
- To reassure patients that there is no reason why they cannot lose weight.
- Height, weight, BMI (>25 overweight, >30 clinically obese), waist circumference (>102 cm for men, >88 cm for women lead to substantially increased health risk), blood pressure, urinalysis, microalbuminuria screen and blood tests if appropriate: consider U&Es TFTs, LFTs, fasting blood glucose, fasting lipids, hormone profile including sex hormones and cortisol. Other tests should be carried out as dictated by comorbidities, e.g. CXR, ECG, glucose tolerance test, HbA_1c, creatinine clearance.
- Bioimpedance analysis (BIA): BMI is an indirect measure of fatness and can be unreliable in e.g. children and athletes. BIA can be used to measure body fat and lean tissue mass; it is reliable and accurate, and can be motivational in patients who become more active and improve their body composition. It is assessed with an inexpensive stand-on body composition analyser.

PRIMARY CARE TEAMWORK

After initial assessment, management should involve as many members of the primary care team as possible, according to availability (including doctors, nurses, dietitian, counsellor, etc.) to provide support and advice about weight loss and its long-term maintenance. Information on local facilities for exercise and physical activity, relevant support groups and weight management groups should be made available. It is essential that each member of the team gives consistent advice, and has a positive approach.

TREATMENT

Parents and families: it is important to give special consideration to situations where parents and other family members are obese or overweight. Parents are important role models for their children, but the child may be the catalyst for change within the whole family. Successful interventions involve the whole family, and the children and/or adolescents, and family should be willing and motivated to make lifestyle changes. Weight maintenance should be addressed at the start of any weight management programme and support for any weight loss achieved should be offered on a long-term basis. Obesity is a chronic condition and its management should be lifelong.

GOALS

Aim for 10% weight loss in 3 months to achieve significant health benefits. 5–10% has also been shown to produce measurable health outcomes. Any weight loss should be encouraged and for some weight maintenance, rather than weight gain may be a realistic goal.

FIRST LINE

The aim is to achieve a 500 kcal deficit of energy requirements through changes in diet and physical activity:

- Support and encouragement, e.g. weight management clinics either within primary care or commercially run.
- Targets, treatments and expectations should be agreed with patients, e.g. 0.5 kg per week, or 10% maintained weight loss rather than 'ideal weight'. Advice about coexisting risk factors, e.g. alcohol, smoking, hyperlipidaemias.
- Regular follow-up appointments with initially monthly, then 1–3 monthly for at least 1 year, to help maintain weight loss.
- Permanent sustainable lifestyle changes: some activity every day; less television, fewer computer games and a less sedentary lifestyle; more exercise; 30–40 minutes sustained exercise, e.g. brisk walking, swimming or cycling, at least 5 days per week.
- More exercise during daily routine; use stairs instead of lifts; walk to work, or park the car further away from work place; take a walk during lunch break. Gardening, washing the car, and activities around the home should be encouraged.
- Encourage activity as a whole family, e.g. walks or trips to the park for relaxation.

DIETARY CHANGES

- Establish regular meals, including breakfast and encourage healthy eating for long term weight management.
- Reduce dietary fat; avoid fried food; encourage grilled, boiled or baked. Buy lean cuts of meat; avoid crisps, pies, cakes, biscuits. Use semi-skimmed milk and low fat spreads.
- Encourage healthy snacks, e.g. fruit as alternatives to sweets, chocolates or crisps.
- Provide advice to patients about food labelling.
- Encourage self-monitoring, i.e. food diaries to enable patient to establish areas for change. Suggested changes need to be tailored to the individual. Giving standard diet sheets is rarely effective.
- Use locally approved advice sheets to ensure consistency of messages. Contact local dietetic departments for guidance.

Other dietary options

- Meal replacements provide a suitable option for some patients. These are structured diet plans normally involving the consumption of two meal replacement drinks per day, plus a self prepared evening meal, fruit and vegetables, totalling approximately 1200–1400 kcal daily. They are purchased from supermarkets and pharmacies.

■ VLCDs (diets containing less than 800 kcal) should only be used under close medical and dietetic supervision.

Success of first-line treatment is gauged after 3–6 months by reduction of BMI, weight reduction (e.g. 5–10% or waist reduction 5–10 cm), improvement of symptoms, or reduced markers of co-morbidity (e.g. exercise tolerance or blood sugar). If these criteria are not achieved, second-line treatment should be considered:

DRUG TREATMENT

■ The pancreatic lipase inhibitor Orlistat may be used in conjunction with a low fat diet to achieve more rapid and greater weight loss. Patients must lose 2.5 kg prior to treatment and demonstrate a 5% reduction in weight in 3 months and 10% in 6 months to comply with licensing and NICE guidelines. It is not absorbed from the gut, and is therefore free from systemic side effects; however patients eating inappropriate high amounts of dietary fat may experience oily bowel motions, flatulence or leakage.

■ Sibutramine inhibits reuptake of serotonin and noradrenaline, which control food intake. It has been shown to be an effective aid to weight reduction and maintenance. It helps patients feel satisfied with smaller portions of food, so that they eat less. It is contraindicated in patients with high or poorly controlled blood pressure (>145/90) or significant cardiovascular disease. BP must be checked initially at 2 weekly intervals for 3 months. Patients must show 2 kg loss at 4 weeks and 5% at 3 months in order to continue treatment.

■ According to their licences and the NICE guidelines, sibutramine and orlistat are indicated for the promotion of weight loss as an adjunctive therapy within a weight management programme for patients with nutritional obesity and a BMI of 30 kg/m² or higher, or for patients with BMI of 28 kg/m² or higher (27 kg/m² for sibutramine), if other obesity-related risk factors are present.

OTHER THERAPIES

■ Behavioural therapy: alternative treatments, including acupuncture and hypnotherapy.

■ Referral to hospital obesity clinic when insufficient weight loss achieved, particularly when BMI >40, or >35 plus comorbidities, or in presence of uncontrolled complications.

■ Bariatric surgery can be extremely successful, but is only indicated in the severely obese; someone who is >100% above their ideal weight, has a BMI >40 or is at immediate risk of serious medical complications. An increasingly common procedure is the laparoscopic gastric band. By this method the functional capacity of the stomach is permanently reduced by the partitioning off of a small segment of the body of the stomach, in order to reduce food intake. Older methods, including the 'Roux-en-Y' technique, surgically bypass the stomach, thereby combining malabsorption of food with restriction of the capacity of the stomach.

An approach to weight management in children and adolescents (2–18 years) in primary care

Produced for the Royal College of Paediatrics and Child Health and National Obesity Forum by Penny Gibson, Laurel Edmunds, David W Haslam, Elizabeth Poskitt.

Overweight children and adolescents can be managed by a primary care team that has a positive attitude to weight management. However the child/adolescent and family should want help and be willing to make lifestyle changes. They may need on-going support to achieve small incremental changes in behaviour. Early intervention is better than waiting until the problem is severe. A sustainable healthy lifestyle is the primary goal of management.

DEFINITIONS AND DIAGNOSIS

Body Mass Index (BMI) is the most practical measure of obesity/overweight, provided values are related to reference standards for age. Currently available British Childhood BMI charts show 91st, 98th and 99.6th centile lines. The 2002 charts also show the recommended International Obesity Task Force cut-offs for obesity and overweight in children. These correspond to the adult definitions of overweight (BMI ≥25) and obesity (BMI ≥30) at age 18. Rapid changes in BMI can occur during normal growth. There is great potential for reducing overweight in childhood and adolescence.

Management decisions depend on:

- the degree of overweight
- age – this influences intervention decisions as well as relative roles of child and family
- related physical or psychological morbidity
- the level of commitment to change, by child and family.

However, the lifestyle approaches described below may be of value to all.

ASSESSMENT

Consider why help is being requested:

- Personal and family history of obesity and related problems e.g. diabetes and CVD. Family structure and social support.

■ Physical activity levels, diet and eating patterns. Consider binge eating disorder and night eating syndrome.
■ Psychological factors leading to or resulting from obesity. Consider self-esteem, bullying, depression, loss or bereavement, sexual abuse etc.
■ Academic progress.

PHYSICAL EXAMINATION

■ Height and weight in light clothing, no shoes. Plot on standard charts with any previous measurements.
■ Features of congenital syndromes, endocrine disorders, learning disability and obesity related morbidities such as orthopaedic problems and sleep apnoea.
■ If acceptable to child/adolescent, evaluate pubertal development.
■ Blood pressure measurement is good practice but requires a suitably sized cuff and table of norms for age.
■ Test urine for glucose and protein.
■ Further investigation should be guided by history and examination, but is seldom required.

INDICATIONS

Indications for possible investigation include short stature, dysmorphic features, severe learning disability, no family history of obesity/overweight.

Rare causes of obesity
■ Endocrine problems (usually have short stature or faltering growth).
■ Hypothyroidism (particularly in Down syndrome).
■ Cushing's syndrome (truncal obesity, hypertension, hirsutism, purple striae).
■ Growth hormone deficiency (may have weight gain and delayed puberty).
■ Chromosomal abnormalities e.g. Prader-Willi (poor linear growth, developmental delay, small genitalia, dysmorphic).
■ Drug related e.g. steroids.

Also predisposing factors such as:

■ spina bifida
■ muscular dystrophy
■ other causes of immobility
■ polycystic ovary syndrome.

REFER TO PAEDIATRICIAN

■ Serious morbidity related to obesity (e.g. sleep apnoea, orthopaedic problems, type 2 and NID diabetes mellitus, hypertension).

- Height below 9th centile, unexpectedly short for family or slowed growth velocity.
- Precocious or late puberty (before 8 years or no signs at 13 in girls, 15 in boys).
- Significant learning disability.
- Symptoms/signs of genetic or endocrine abnormalities.
- Severe and progressive obesity before age 2.
- Other significant concerns.

WEIGHT MANAGEMENT OPTIONS
- No weight gain as height increases.
- Weight gain slower than height gain.

NB: Rapid weight loss and strict dieting are not appropriate for growing children unless under specialist care. Children over 7 years old with obesity and/or complications may benefit from gradual weight loss e.g. 0.5 kg/month. If adolescents have stopped growing, weight loss of around 0.5 kg/week may be appropriate.

ACTION
Successful interventions involve the family and are tailored to each individual. Parents are important role models, particularly for younger children. Weight gain is controlled by addressing eating habits, physical activity and inactivity, psychosocial and family issues.

The multidisciplinary team needed may include GP, Practice Nurse, Health Visitor, School Nurse and other professionals if available e.g. Paediatric Dietician, Clinical Psychologist, Community Paediatrician.

PHYSICAL ACTIVITY SUGGESTIONS
- Any increase in activity will help.
- Aim for sustainable lifestyle activity such as walking, cycling, using the stairs instead of lifts.
- Develop an active lifestyle in the whole family.
- Walk or cycle to school.
- Encourage active play that is enjoyable and activities that do not cause embarrassment.
- Decrease TV viewing and other sedentary behaviours.

DIETARY SUGGESTIONS
- A balanced, varied diet for the whole family.
- Meals at regular times; avoid grazing and TV snacks.
- Smaller portions.
- Avoid using food/snacks as rewards or treats.

- Healthy snacks (e.g. fruit) as alternatives to sweets, chocolates, crisps, nuts, biscuits, cakes.
- Less energy-dense food, e.g. semi-skimmed milks, low fat spreads.
- Wholefoods, which take time to eat e.g. fruits and wholemeal bread.
- At least 5 portions of fruit and vegetables per day.
- Low-calorie drinks (preferably water).
- Grill, boil or bake foods without added fat, rather than frying.
- Negotiate realistic goals and monitoring plans. Parents should be involved as much as possible, but adolescents may prefer to take responsibility for themselves.
- Make small, progressive, sustainable changes in eating habits, physical activity and inactivity.
- Develop coping strategies for teasing/bullying and steps to increase self-esteem and confidence.
- Address psychosocial issues. Consider using counselling or specialist services.
- Encourage positive parenting styles that will develop emotional well being. Involve Health Visitor and use parenting education and support as appropriate.
- Offer regular follow up, e.g. weekly initially, then monthly.

Make available information on:

- local physical activity facilities.
- healthy eating.
- local parenting support groups.

Keep a positive attitude! Always consider the feelings and sensitivities of each child or adolescent.

To be read in conjunction with the childhood guidelines

An approach to weight management in children and adolescents (2–18 years) in primary care provides advice to professionals about the management of overweight and obesity. The working group members are:

- Dr Penny Gibson – Consultant Paediatrician and RCPCH advisor on Childhood Obesity.
- Dr Laurel Edmunds – Research Fellow, University of Oxford, researching childhood obesity.
- Dr David W Haslam – GP and Vice Chairman of National Obesity Forum.
- Dr Elizabeth Poskitt – Paediatrician and Honorary Senior Lecturer in Nutrition, London School of Hygiene.

The management of obesity is complex. We need more evidence and look forward to seeing the results of current and future research. However there is already an extensive literature, which has been reviewed and used in the development of this advice. Between June and December 2001, the working group drafted a document for use in primary care. We then used extensive consultation in order to develop a pragmatic and practical approach.

We were aware of the development of guidelines by SIGN – *Obesity in children and young people. A national clinical guideline*. We have compared our advice with the draft SIGN document and feel it is compatible and complementary.

The draft document was widely circulated for consultation to members of:

- the known network of academics and practitioners in the field
- National Obesity Forum (NOF)
- RCPCH
- Association for the Study of Obesity (ASO)
- TOAST
- RCGP
- RCN
- CPHVA
- BDA
- Child Public Health Interest Group of RCPCH and FPHM
- All delegates at the National Audit Office meeting 'Joining forces to tackle obesity' in January 2002
- Department of Health
- Health Development Agency
- Others.

We received over 50 responses from doctors, nurses, dietitians, academics and parents.

The working group reviewed and altered the document before obtaining final comments and approval from the RCPCH Nutrition committee and Executive Council.

The document has been distributed to all GPs via the *GP* magazine (April/May 2002) and to all members of RCPCH (June 2002), with attached copies of BMI charts. Electronic versions will be sent to other organizations and individuals.

Our work has been supported and facilitated by the RCPCH, NOF, Department of Health, Child Growth Foundation, Harlow Printing and *GP* magazine.

Please contact Dr Penny Gibson (penny.gibson@shb-tr.nhs.uk) for further information or comments. We would welcome research or audit ideas and help, related to this advice.

The following references[1–16] include review papers used as part of the evidence base for the 'Approach' and other papers of interest.

References

1. The prevention and treatment of obesity: NHS Centre for Reviews and Dissemination, University of York, 1997 3(2):1–12.
2. Barlow SE, Dietz WH. Obesity evaluation and treatment: Expert Committee recommendations. Pediatrics 1998 102(3):E29.
3. Beck S, Terry K. A comparison of obese and normal-weight families' psychological characteristics. American Journal of Family Therapy 1985 13(3):55–59.
4. Campbell K, Waters E, O'Meara S, Summerbell C. Interventions for preventing obesity in children (Cochrane Review). Cochrane Database System Review 2001 2:CD001871.
5. Cole TJ, Bellizzi MC, Flegal KM, Dietz WH. Establishing a standard definition for child overweight and obesity worldwide: international survey. British Medical Journal 2000 320(7244):1240–1243.
6. Edmunds L, Waters E. Childhood obesity. In: Moyer VA et al (eds). Evidence-based pediatrics and child health. BMJ Press, London, 2000, p 141–156.
7. Epstein LH, Goldfield GS. Physical activity in the treatment of childhood overweight and obesity: current evidence and research issues. Medicine and Science in Sports and Exercise 1999 31(11 suppl):S553–S559.
8. Epstein LH, Myers MD, Raynor HA, Saelens BE. Treatment of pediatric obesity. Pediatrics 1998 101(suppl):554–570.
9. Gill TP. Key issues in the prevention of obesity. British Medical Bulletin 1997 53(2):359–388.
10. French SA, Story M, Perry CL. Self-esteem and obesity in children and adolescents: a literature review. Obesity Research 1995 3(5):479–490.
11. Glenny AM, O'Meara S, Melville A, Sheldon TA, Wilson C. The treatment and prevention of obesity: a systematic review of the literature. International Journal of Obesity and Related Metabolic Disorders 1997 21(9):715–737.
12. Haddock CK, Shadish WR, Klesges RC, Stein RJ. Treatments for childhood and adolescent obesity. Annals of Behavioral Medicine 1994 16(3):235–244.
13. Hardeman W, Griffin S, Johnston M, Kinmonth AL, Wareham NJ. Interventions to prevent weight gain: a systematic review of psychological models and behaviour change methods. International Journal of Obesity 2000 24(2):131–143.
14. Jebb S. The weight of the nation. Obesity in the UK. MRC Human Nutrition Research, London.
15. Jelalian E, Saelens BE. Empirically supported treatments in pediatric psychology: pediatric obesity. Journal of Pediatric Psychology 1999 24(3):223–248.
16. Parsons TJ, Power C, Logan S, Summerbell CD. Childhood predictors of adult obesity: a systematic review. International Journal of Obesity 1999 23(suppl 8):S1–S107.

National Obesity Forum pharmacotherapy guidelines for obesity management in adults

CHOICE OF ANTIOBESITY AGENT

There are two agents currently available for pharmacotherapy as part of a weight management programme for obese and overweight patients; orlistat and sibutramine. There is no evidence that bulking agents such as methylcellulose or ispaghula husk have any role to play in long-term weight management. Metformin can be an effective drug for weight management in diabetic patients, and its effect on insulin resistance has been utilized in obese non-diabetic subjects to aid weight loss, but it should not be prescribed for this purpose in primary care. Unlicensed drugs including phentermine and diethylpropion have no place in pharmacotherapy of obesity and have profound safety implications. However they are still prescribed by some sources, and may be encountered in primary care.

Orlistat and sibutramine exhibit different pharmacological profiles, contraindications and side-effects.

NICE Guidance and the SPC Product Licenses for both products have differences with regard to eligibility of drug treatment, requirements prior to starting therapy and continuation of therapy. They cannot be used together.

COMPARISON OF ORLISTAT AND SIBUTRAMINE ELIGIBILITY (SPC AND NICE)

Eligibility for treatment initiation

	Orlistat (Xenical)	Sibutramine (Reductil)
BMI over 30	✔	✔
BMI over 27 + comorbidity	–	✔
BMI over 28 + comorbidity	✔	✔

Comorbidities include diabetes, hyperlipidaemia and hypertension.

CHD and stroke may also be included under the heading of 'comorbidity' for orlistat.

Sibutramine is contraindicated if blood pressure is not controlled at <145/90 mmHg.

PRE-THERAPY REQUIREMENTS PRIOR TO RECEIVING 1ST PRESCRIPTION
- Orlistat (Xenical): patient is required to display weight loss of at least 2.5kg through lifestyle.
- Sibutramine (Reductil): patient has been unable to display weight loss of at least 5% through lifestyle change within the last 3 months.

CONTINUATION OF THERAPY

	Orlistat (Xenical)	Sibutramine (Reductil)
2-week criteria BP		Check fortnightly
1-month criteria		2-kg weight loss
3-month criteria	5% weight loss	5% weight loss
6-month criteria	10% weight loss	10% weight loss
Current cost (1 year of treatment)	£537 (1 capsule 3 times daily)	£456–£510 (10–15 mg once daily)

Evidence shows that maintaining 5% weight loss is clinically beneficial.

POPULATIONS WHERE DRUGS ARE CONTRAINDICATED
- Preconception, pregnancy or breast-feeding children (under 18 years).
- Elderly (over 65 years) BMI <27.
- Significant drug interactions.

DRUGS THAT MAY CAUSE WEIGHT GAIN
- Antipsychotics: especially olanzepine (Zyprexa).
- Antidepressants: tricyclics, SSRIs, MAOIs and mirtazepine (Zispin), and lithium.
- Corticosteroids: all corticosteroids may promote weight gain by two mechanisms: fat redistribution causing truncal obesity, buffalo hump and moon face, and fluid retention via mineralocorticoid effects.
- OCP: progestogenic compounds.
- β-blockers: not only do these agents cause weight gain, they may restrict physical activity due to fatigue.
- Oral hypoglycaemics: Numerous agents shown to increase weight. Most sulphonylureas (except glimepiride). Glitazones.
- Insulin.
- Anticonvulsants: weight gain has been documented with some agents (phenytoin, sodium valproate). Topiramate (Topamax) is weight neutral or may cause weight loss.
- Antihistamines: many antihistamines may cause weight gain though these effects are more pronounced with older agents.

Orlistat (Xenical)

Orlistat promotes weight loss by reducing the absorption of energy dense fat. It is a potent inhibitor of pancreatic and gastric lipases, which are enzymes responsible for breaking down fat, allowing approximately 30% of dietary fat to pass through the GI tract unabsorbed.

DOSAGE, SIDE-EFFECTS AND CONTRAINDICATIONS

- One capsule (120 mg) before, during or up to 1 hour after main meal, up to 3 times a day.
- Dose can be missed if meal is missed.
- ADR: oily spotting with flatus, faecal urgency and anal leakage (if inappropriate diet is consumed).
- Patients on orlistat should adhere to a diet that is nutritionally balanced, mildly hypocaloric and contains less than 30% of calories from fat.

SPECIAL WARNINGS AND CONTRAINDICATIONS

- Rarely, malabsorption of fat soluble vitamins (A, D, E and K) may occur, although this is not an issue for the majority of patients in primary care.
- Physicians may choose to supplement those who are on therapy for longer than 1 year.
- Orlistat is contraindicated in patients with cholestasis or malabsorptive syndromes.
- There is no evidence to associate orlistat with increase in breast cancer.

DRUG INTERACTIONS

- Treatment with orlistat may reduce the absorption of ciclosporin – monitor blood levels.
- Treatment with orlistat may reduce vitamin K absorption – always monitor INR on warfarin patients.

PATIENT CONSIDERATIONS FOR DISCUSSION

- GI side-effects may reduce compliance if patient is not forewarned.
- Some patients learn which food types give them side-effects and modify their diets to reduce these.
- Some patients may choose to omit doses when dining out or eating fatty food; discuss with patient.
- Patients who supplement multi-vitamins should leave a 2-hour gap either side of orlistat dosing.

Patients on orlistat may be encouraged to contact the Medical Action Plan helpline supported by Roche: 0800 731 7138.

Sibutramine (Reductil)

Sibutramine is not an appetite suppressant. It inhibits the reuptake of both serotonin and noradrenaline in the brain. Weight loss is mediated via two mechanisms. Firstly, sibutramine's central action on neurotransmitters results in early satiety (feeling of fullness) with reported 20% reduction in food intake. Secondly, sympathetically mediated thermogenesis maintains original basal metabolic rate (BMR), which usually falls as weight is lost. This results in energy expenditure and contributes to further weight loss.

DOSAGE, SIDE-EFFECTS AND CONTRAINDICATIONS

- One 10-mg capsule once daily. This may be increased to a maximum of 15 mg once daily.
- Increase from 10 mg to 15 mg daily should be considered at 1 month if less than 2 kg has been lost.
- ADR: headache, dizziness, sweating, palpitations, constipation and dry mouth.

CONTRAINDICATIONS

Sibutramine should not be used in the following situations:

- History of CHD, cardiac arrhythmias or uncontrolled hypertension.
- History of stroke or heart failure.
- History of eating disorders or psychiatric illness.
- Patients on antipsychotics or antidepressants.

The European Committee for Proprietary Medicinal Products (CPMP) has investigated sibutramine and concluded that it exhibits a positive favourable risk profile for the management of obesity (May 2002).

Sibutramine can be used safely in hypertensives who are well controlled (BP not over 145/90 mmHg):

- Patients require pulse and blood pressure monitoring (every 2 weeks for 3 months, then every 4 weeks for 3 months, then every 3 months thereafter).
- STOP THERAPY: if blood pressure rises by 10 mmHg, two readings.
- STOP THERAPY: if pulse rises by 10 beats per minute.
- INVESTIGATE reports of breathing problems, palpitations or chest pain.

PATIENT CONSIDERATIONS FOR DISCUSSION

- Sibutramine should only be used in conjunction with appropriate lifestyle changes to diet and physical activity.
- The satiety effect of this agent should be emphasized – expect to eat less at meals; encourage the use of smaller plates and portion sizes, and reduce snacking.

- Most patients on sibutramine actually show reductions in BP. Reassure the patient of this.
- Non-responders to sibutramine are more likely to show increases in blood pressure.
- The SPC confirms the incidence of patients experiencing blood pressure increase is less than 10%.
- Patients should be cautioned on use of OTC decongestants (sympathomimetics) as they may increase BP.

Patients on sibutramine may be encouraged to contact the Change for Life programme supported by Abbott: 0800 389 4669.

REFERENCES

Chapter 1

National Center for Health Statistics 2003 Third National Health and Nutrition Examination Survey (NHANES III, 1988–1994). Centers for Disease Control and Prevention, Washington DC. Online. Available: www.xenical.com/hcp/2_hromr.asp

Reilly JJ, Dorosty AR 1999 Epidemic of obesity in UK children. Lancet 354:1874–1875

World Health Organization 1997 Obesity: preventing and managing the global epidemic. WHO Technical Report Series, No. 894. Geneva, World Health Organization. Online. Available: www.who.int/nut/publications.htm

Chapter 2

Allied Dunbar 1992 National Fitness Survey: a report on activity patterns and fitness levels. Sports Council and Health Education Authority, London

Almond L, Newberry I 2000 The importance of physical activity in weight management. Obesity in Practice 2(2):10–12

American Diabetes Association 2003 63rd Scientific sessions, July 2003. Online. Available: medscape (www.medscape.com)

British Nutrition Foundation (BNF)Task Force Report 1999 Obesity. Blackwell, London

Blair S, Kohl H, Gordon N 1992 Physical activity and health: a lifestyle approach. Medicine Exercise Nutrition and Health 1: 54–7

Bundred P, Kitchiner D, Buchan I 2001 Prevalence of overweight and obese children between 1989 and 1998: population based series of cross sectional studies. BMJ 10;322(7282):326–8

Considine RV, Sinha MK, Heiman ML et al 1996 Serum immunoreactive leptin concentrations in normal-weight and obese humans. New England Journal of Medicine 334:292–295

Engeli S, Feldpausch M, Gorzelniak K et al 2003 Association between adiponectin and mediators of inflammation in obese women. Diabetes 52:942–947. Online. Available: www.medscape.com

Maes HH et al 1997 Genetic and environmental factors in relative body weight and human adiposity. Behavior Genetics 27:325–351

National Audit Office 2002 Tackling obesity in England. Report by the comptroller and auditor general. HC 220, Session 2000–2001. 15 February 2001, para 2.15

Samaras K et al 1999 Genetic and environmental influences on total body-fat and central abdominal fat. Annals of Internal Medicine 130:873–882

Steppan CM et al 2001 The hormone resistin links obesity to diabetes. Nature 409(6818):207–212

Ukkola O 2002 Resistin – a mediator of obesity-associated insulin resistance or an innocent bystander? European Journal of Endocrinology 147(5):571–574

Waine C 2002 Obesity and weight management in primary care. Blackwell Science, Oxford, p 12

Yang R, Xu A, Pray J et al 2003 Cloning of omentin, a new adipocytokine from omental fat tissue in humans. Program and abstracts of the 63rd Scientific Session of the American Diabetes Association; June 13–17, 2003; New

Orleans, LA. Abstract 1-OR. Online. Available: www.medscape.com/viewarticle/458393

Chapter 3

Adams JP, Murphy PG 2000 Obesity in anaesthesia and intensive care. British Journal of Anaesthesiology 85: 91–108

American Academy of Allergy, Asthma and Immunology 2003 Annual Meeting, Denver, 7–12 March 2003

Baeten JM, Bukusi EA, Lambe M 2001 Pregnancy complications and outcomes among overweight and obese nulliparous women. American Journal of Public Health 91:436–440

Blackburn G 1995 Effect of degree of weight loss on health benefits. Obesity Research 3(suppl 2):211s–216s.

British Nutrition Foundation (BNF) Task Force Report 1999 Obesity. Blackwell, London

Bremer JM, Scott RS, Lintott CJ 1994 Dexfenfluramine reduces cardiovascular risk factors. International Journal of Obesity-related Metabolic Disorders 18:199–205

Brenner JS, Kelly CS, Wenger AD et al 2001 Asthma and obesity in adolescents: is there an association? Journal of Asthma 38(6):509–515.

Calandra C, Abell DA, Beischer NA 1981 Maternal obesity in pregnancy. Obstetrics and Gynecology 57:8

Camargo CA, Weiss ST, Zhang S et al 1999 Prospective study of body mass index, weight change, and risk of adult-onset asthma in women. Archives of Internal Medicine 159:2582–2588

Cassano PA, Segal MR, Vokonas PS et al 1990 Body fat distribution, blood pressure, and hypertension. A prospective cohort study of men in the normative aging study. Annals of Epidemiology 1:33–48

Chambers R et al 2000 Weight loss, weight maintenance and improved cardiac risk factors after 2 years of treatment with orlistat for obesity. Obesity Research 8:49–61

Chan JM, Stampler MJ, Rimm EB et al 1994 Obesity, fat distribution and weight gain as risk factors for clinical diabetes in man. Diabetes Care 17, 961–969.

Checkley E 1892 A natural method of physical training. William C. Bryant, New York, p 89.

Chinn S, Rona RJ 2001 Can the increase in body mass index explain the rising trend in asthma in children? Thorax 56(11):845–850.

Choi HK, Atkinson K, Karlson EW, Curhan G. Weight gain, obesity, and incident gout in a large, long-term, prospective cohort study. Program and abstracts of the American College of Rheumatology 66th Annual Scientific Meeting; October 25–29, 2002. New Orleans. LA. Abstract 1593

Chow W-H, Gridley G, Fraumeni JF, Järvholm B 2000 Obesity, hypertension, and the risk of kidney cancer in men. New England Journal of Medicine 343(18):1305–1311.

Cicuttini FM, Baker JR, Spector TD 1996 The association of obesity with osteoarthritis of the hand and knee in women: a twin study. Journal of Rheumatology 23(7):1221–1226.

Colditz G, Willett W, Stampfer M et al 1990 Patterns of weight gain and their relation to diet in a cohort of healthy women. American Journal of Clinical Nutrition 51:1100–1105

Colditz GA, Willett WC, Rotnitzkya A, Manson JE 1995 Weight gain as a risk factor for clinical diabetes. Annals of Internal Medicine 122(7):481–486

Coleman RM, Roffwarg HP, Kennedy SJ et al 1982 Sleep wake disorders based on polysomnographic diagnosis. A national cooperative study. Journal of the American Medical Association 247:997–1003

Davies RJ, Stradling JR 1990 The relationship between neck circumference, radiographic pharyngeal anatomy, and the obstructive sleep apnoea syndrome. European Respiratory Journal 3:509–514

Day CP 2002 Non-alcoholic steatohepatitis (NASH): where are we now and where are we going? Gut 50:585–588

de Knegt RJ 2001 Non-alcoholic steatohepatitis: clinical significance and pathogenesis. Scandinavian Journal of Gastroenterology suppl 234:88–92

Edwards LE, Dickes WF, Alton IR et al 1978 Pregnancy in the massively obese. Course, outcome, and obesity prognosis of the infant. American Journal of Obstetrics and Gynecology 131:479

Egan BM 2003 Insulin resistance and the sympathetic nervous system. Current Hypertension Reports 5(3):247–254

Felson DT, Anderson JJ, Naimark A et al 1988 Obesity and knee osteoarthritis. The Framingham Study. Annals of Internal Medicine 109(1):18–24. Online. Available: www.ncbi.nlm.nih.gov

Ford ES, Williamson DF, Liu S 1997 Weight change and diabetes incidence: findings from a cohort of US adults. American Journal of Epidemiology 146:214–222

Fujioka K, Seaton TB, Rowe E et al and the Diabetes Clinical Study Group 2000 Weight loss with sibutramine improves glycaemic control and other metabolic parameters in obese patients with type 2 diabetes mellitus. Diabetes, Obesity and Metabolism 2(3):175–187

Galtier-Dereure F, Boegner C, Bringer J 2000 Obesity and pregnancy: complications and cost. American Journal of Clinical Nutrition 71:1242S

Gannong W 1999 Review of medical physiology, 19th ed. Appleton and Lange, New York, p 519.

Garbaciak JA, Richter M, Miller S, et al 1985 Maternal weight and pregnancy complications. American Journal of Obstetrics and Gynecology 152:238

Garfinkel L 1985 Overweight and cancer. Annals of Internal Medicine 103:1034–1036.

Green BB, Weiss NB, Daling JR 1988 Risk of ovulatory infertility in relation to body weight. Fertility and Sterility 50:721

Havlik RJ, Hubert HB, Fabsitz RR, Feinleib M 1983 Weight and hypertension. Annals of Internal Medicine 98(pt 2):855–859

Hendricks KA, Nuno OM, Suarez L, Larsen R 2001 Effects of hyperinsulinemia and obesity on risk of neural tube defects among Mexican Americans. Epidemiology 12:630

Herbert H, Fernlab M, McNamara P et al 1983 Obesity as an independent risk factor for cardiovascular disease. A 26-year follow- up of participants in the Framingham Study. Circulation 67:968–977

Jordan KM, Dennison EM, Syddall H, Arden NK, Cooper C 2002 Birthweight and spinal osteoarthritis: evidence for intrauterine programming. Program and abstracts of the American College of Rheumatology 66th Annual Scientific Meeting; October 25–29. New Orleans, LA. Abstract 1238

Jung R 1997 Obesity as a disease. British Medical Bulletin 53:307–321

Khedr M, Elias E 2003 Non-alcoholic fatty liver disease: can weight loss help? Obesity in Practice 5(1):12–15.

Kumari AS 2001 Pregnancy outcome in women with morbid obesity. International Journal of Gynecology and Obstetrics 73:101

Lavie C, Ventura H, Messerli F 1992 Left ventricular hypertrophy. Its relationship to obesity and hypertension. Postgraduate Medicine 91:131–143

Lethbridge-Cejku M, Creamer P, Scott WW Jr, Ling SM, Metter J, Hochberg MC 2002 Weight loss is associated with reduced risk of incident radiographic knee osteoarthritis in men but not in women: data from the Baltimore Longitudinal Study of Aging. Program and abstracts of the American College of Rheumatology 66th Annual Scientific Meeting; October 25–29. New Orleans, LA. Abstract 1235

McMahon S, Cutler J, Brittain E et al 1987 Obesity and hypertension: epidemiological and clinical issues. European Heart Journal 8(suppl B):57–70

Meade TW, Ruddock V, Stirling Y et al 1993 Fibrinolytic activity, clotting factors and long-term incidence of ischaemic heart disease in the Northwick Park study. Lancet 342:1076–1079

National Center for Health Statistics 2003 Third National Health and Nutrition Examination Survey (NHANES III, 1988–1994). Centers for Disease Control and Prevention, Washington DC. Online. Available: www.xenical.com/hcp/2_hromr.asp

Norman R et al 2001 Announced at European Society of Human Reproduction and Embryology (ESHRE), Lausanne 2 July 2001. Online. Available: www.eshre.com

Olson C 2001 Excessive weight gain during pregnancy: a major contributor to obesity. January 2001. Online. Available: www.pslgroup.com/dg/1F07FE.htm

Pi-Sunyer FX 1993 Medical hazards of obesity. Annals of Internal Medicine 119(7 pt 2):655–660

Rooney BL & Schauberger CW 2002 Excess pregnancy weight gain and long-term obesity: one decade later. Obstetrics and Gynaecology 100(2):245–252

Rossner S, Sjostrum L, Noack R et al 2000 Weight loss, weight maintenance and improved cardiac risk factors after 2 years of treatment with orlistat for obesity. Obesity Research 8:49–61

Shaper AG, Phillips AN, Pocock SJ et al 1991 Risk factors for stroke in middle aged British men. BMJ 302:1111–1115.

Shiffman ML, Sugerman HJ, Kellum JM, Moore EW 1992 Changes in gallbladder bile composition following gallstone formation and weight reduction. Gastroenterology 103(1)214–221.

Sims EAH, Danforth E Horton ES et al 1973 Endocrine and metabolic effects of experimental obesity in man. Recent Progress in Hormone Research 29:457–496

Sin DD, Jones RL, Man SFP 2002 Obesity is a risk factor for dyspnea but not for airflow obstruction. Archives of Internal Medicine 162:1477–1481

Spitzer RL, Yanovski S, Wadden T, Wing R, Marcus MD, Stunkard A et al 1993 Binge eating disorder: its further validation in a multisite study. International Journal of Eating Disorders 13(2):137–153

Stickles B, Phillips L, Brox WT et al 2001 Defining the relationship between obesity and total joint arthroplasty. Obesity Research 9(3):219–223.

Stoohs RA, Guilleminault C, Itoi A, Dement WC 1994 Traffic accidents in commercial long-haul truck drivers: the influence of sleep-disordered breathing and obesity. Sleep 17(7):619–623.

Suk SH, Sacco RL, Boden-Albala B et al 2003 Abdominal obesity and risk of ischemic stroke: the Northern Manhattan Stroke Study. Stroke 34(7):1586–1592.

Trent JT, Kirsner RS 2002 Diagnosing necrotizing fasciitis. Advances in Skin Wound Care 15(3):135–138.

van Saase JL, Vandenbroucke JP, van Romunde LK, Valkenburg HA. 1988 Osteoarthritis and obesity in the general population. A relationship calling for an explanation. Journal of Rheumatology 15(7):1152–1158

Vaughan RW, Engelhardt RC, Wise L 1976 Postoperative hypoxemia in obese patients. Annals of Surgery 180:877

Vazquez-Vela Johnson G, Worland R L, Keenan J, Norambuena N 2003 Patient demographics as a predictor of the ten-year survival rate in primary total knee replacement. Journal of Bone and Joint Surgery 85(1):52–56.

von Kries R, Toschke AM, Koletzko B, Slikker S Jr 2002 Maternal smoking during pregnancy and childhood obesity. American Journal of Epidemiology 156:954–961

von Mutius E, Schwartz J, Neas LM et al 2001 Relation of body mass index to asthma and atopy in children: the National Health and Nutrition Examination Study III. Thorax 56(11):835–838

Waine C 2002 Obesity and weight management in primary care. Blackwell Science, Oxford, p 36

Weintraub M, Sundaresan PR, Madan M, et al 1992 Long-term weight control study I (weeks 0 to 34). The enhancement of behaviour modification, caloric restriction, and exercise by fenfluramine plus phentermine versus placebo. Clinical Pharmacology and Therapeutics 51:586–594

Whiteman MK, Staropoli CA, Langenberg PW et al 2003 Smoking, body mass, and hot flashes in midlife women. Potentially modifiable factors, such as current smoking and high body mass index, may predispose a woman to more severe or frequent hot flashes. Obstetrics and Gynecology 101(2):264–272

Williamson DF, Pamuk E, Thun M et al 1995 Prospective study of intentional weight loss and mortality in never-smoking overweight US white women aged 40–64 years. American Journal of Epidemiology 141:1128–1141.

Wolf AM, Colditz GA. Current estimates of the economic cost of obesity in the United States. Obesity Research 1998 6:97–106.

Wolk A, Gridley G, Svensson M et al 2001 A prospective study of obesity and cancer risk (Sweden). Cancer Causes and Control 12(1):13–21.

World Health Organization 1997 Obesity: preventing and managing the global epidemic. WHO Technical Report Series, No. 894. Geneva, World Health Organization. Online. Available www.who.int/nut/publications.htm

World Health Organization, Regional Office for the Western Pacific, International Association for the study of obesity 2000 International Obesity Task Force. The Asia-Pacific perspective: redefining obesity and its treatment. Melbourne: Health Communications Australia

Chapter 4

Ackard DM, Neumark-Sztainer D, Story M, Perry C 2003 Overeating among adolescents: prevalence and associations with weight-related characteristics and psychological health. Pediatrics 111:67–74.

American Journal of Physiology, Endocrinology and Metabolism 2002 282:E366–E369

American Journal of Public Health 2000 90:251–271

Birketvedt GS, Sundsfjord J, Florholmen JR 2002 Hypothalamic-pituitary-adrenal axis in the night eating syndrome. American Journal of Physiology, Endocrinology and Metabolism 282:E366–E369.

British Nutrition Foundation (BNF) Task Force Report 1999 Obesity. Blackwell, London

Carpenter KM, Hasin DS, Allison DB, Faith MS 2000 Relationships between obesity and DSM-IV major depressive disorder, suicide ideation, and suicide attempts: results from a general population study. American Journal of Public Health 90:251–257.

Dunea G 1997 Magna meno (Eat less). British Medical Journal 314:7075

Galasko D 2003 Insulin and Alzheimer's disease: an amyloid connection. Neurology 60:1886–1887.

Gortmaker SL, Must A, Perrin JM et al 1993 Social and economic consequences of overweight in adolescence and young adulthood. New England Journal of Medicine 329:1008–1012.

Johnson LN Krohel GB, March GA Jr. 1999 Author's reply to Pomeranz HD: Weight loss, acetazolamide, and pseudotumor cerebri [letter]. Ophthalmology 106:1639.

Lindroos A-K, Lissner L, Sjostrom L 1996 Weight change in relation to intake of sugar and sweet foods before and after weight reducing gastric surgery. International Journal of Obesity 20:634–643.

Lissau I, Sorensen TIA 1994 Parental neglect during childhood and increased risk of obesity in young adulthood. Lancet 343:324–327.

Pine DS, Goldstein RB, Wolk S, Weissman MM 2001 The association between childhood depression and adulthood body mass index. Pediatrics 107:1049–1056.

Roberts RE, Strawbridge WJ, Deleger S, Kaplan GA 2002 Are the fat more jolly? Annals of Behavioural Medicine 24(3):169–180.

Rothschild M, Peterson HR, Pfeifer MA 1989 Depression in obese men. International Journal of Obesity 13:479–485.

Schenck CH, Mahowald MW 1994 Review of nocturnal sleep-related eating disorders. International Journal of Eating Disorders 15:343–356.

Seddon JM, Cote J, Davis N, Rosner B 2003 Progression of age-related macular degeneration: association with body mass index, waist circumference, and waist-hip ratio. Archives of Ophthalmology 121(6):785–792

Spitzer RL, Yanovski S, Wadden T, Wing R, Marcus MD, Stunkard A et al 1993 Binge eating disorder: its further validation in a multisite study. International Journal of Eating Disorders 13(2):137–153

Stunkard AJ 1980 Pain of obesity. Bull Publishing Co, California, p 75.

Volkow ND, Wang G-J, Fowler JS et al 2002 Nonhedonic food motivation in humans involves dopamine in the dorsal striatum and methylphenidate amplifies this effect. Synapse 44(3).

Wadden TA, Foster GD, Stunkard AJ, Linowitz JR 1989 Dissatisfaction with weight and figure in obese girls; discontent but not depression. International Journal of Obesity 13:89–97.

Chapter 5

Jung RT 1997 Obesity as a disease. British Medical Bulletin 53(2):307–21

Oster G et al 1999 Lifetime health and economic benefits of weight loss among obese persons. American Journal of Public Health 89:1536–1542

Walker A 2003 The Cost of Doing Nothing - the economics of obesity in Scotland. Online. Available: www.scottish.parliament.uk

Chapter 6

Al-Zahrani MS, Bissada NF, Borawskit EA 2003 Obesity and periodontal disease in young, middle-aged, and older adults. Journal of Periodontology 74(5):610–615.

Arbuthnot J 1735 An essay concerning the nature of ailments, 3rd edn. Tonson, London, p 196

Armstrong N, Balding J, Gentle P, Kirby P, 1990 Patterns of physical activity among 11–16-year-old British children. British Medican Journal 301:203–205.

Baker LC, Kirschenbaum DS 1993 Self-monitoring may be necessary for successful weight reduction. Behaviour Therapy 24:377–394.

Ballor DL, Poehlman ET 1994 Exercise-training enhances fat-free mass preservation during diet-induced weight loss: a meta-analytical finding. International Journal of Obesity 18:35–40.

Blundell JE, King NA 1998 Effects of exercise on appetite control: loose coupling between energy expenditure and energy intake. International Journal of Obesity 22(suppl2):S22–S29.

British Nutrition Foundation (BNF) Task Force Report 1999 Obesity. Blackwell, London

Brownell KD 1997 The Learn programme for weight control. American Health Publishing Company, Dallas, TX

Capstick F, Brooks BA, Burns CM et al 1997 Very low calorie diets (VLCD): a useful alternative in the treatment of the obese NIDDM patient. Diabetes Research and Clinical Practice 36(2):105–111.

Costain L 2003 Diet trials. BBC Publications, London, p 204

Crespo CH, Smit E, Troiano RP et al 2001 Television watching, energy intake and obesity in US children: results from the third National Health and Nutrition Examination Survey 1988–1994. Archives of Pediatric and Adolescent Medicine 115:360–365.

Ditschuneit HH, Flechtner-Mors M, Johnson TD, Adler G 1989 Metabolic and weight-loss effects of a long-term dietary intervention in obese patients. American Journal of Clinical Nutrition 69(2):198–204.

Ditschuneit HH, Frier HI, Flechtner-Mors M 2002 Lipoprotein responses to weight loss and weight maintenance in high-risk obese subjects. European Journal of Clinical Nutrition 56(3):264–270.

Epstein LH, Valoski AM, Vara LS et al 1995 Effects of decreasing sedentary behaviour and increasing activity on weight changes in obese children. Health Psychology 14:1–7.

Ferster CD, Nurnberger JI, Levitt EB. 1962 The control of eating. Journal of Mathematics 1:87–109.

Garrow JS, Webster JD, Pearson M et al 1989 Inpatient-outpatient randomised comparison of the Cambridge diet versus milk diet in 17 obese women over 24 weeks. International Journal of Obesity 13:521–529.

Garrow J 1999 Obesity. British Nutrition Foundation, London, p 164.

Garrow JS, Summerbell CD 1995 Meta-analysis: effect of exercise, with or without dieting, on body composition of overweight subjects. European Journal of Clinical Nutrition 49:1–10.

Gately PJ, Cooke CB 2003 A residential summer camp programme for the treatment of obese and overweight children. Obesity in Practice 5(1):2–5.

Gilman Thompson W 1909 Practical dietetics. Appleton, New York.

Gortmaker SL, Must A, Sobol AM et al 1996 Television viewing as a cause of increasing obesity among children in the United States 1986–90. Archives of Pediatric and Adolescent Medicine 150:356–362.

Health Education Authority 1991 Health and lifestyle survey. HEA, London.

Helmrich SP, Ragland DR, Leung RW, Paffenbarger RS Jr 1991 Physical activity and reduced occurrence of non-insulin-dependent diabetes mellitus. New England Journal of Medicine 325(3):147–152.

Krotkiewski M, Mandroukas K, Sjostrom L et al 1979 Effects of long-term physical training on body fat, metabolism, and blood pressure in obesity. Metabolism 28(6):650–658.

Lee CD, Jackson AS, Blair SN 1998 US weight guidelines: is it also important to consider cardio-respiratory fitness? International Journal of Obesity 22(suppl 20):S2–S7.

Morgan WP 1997 Physical activity and mental health. Taylor and Francis, Washington DC, pp 93–106, 107–127.

National Audit Office 2002 Tackling obesity in England. Report by the comptroller and auditor general. HC 220, Session 2000–2001. 15 February 2001, para 2.13.

National Task Force for Prevention and Treatment of Obesity 1993 Very low-calorie diets. Objective: to provide an overview of the published scientific information on the safety and efficacy of very low-calorie diets (VLCDs) and to provide rational recommendations for their use. Journal of the American Medical Association 270:967–974.

Paylou KN, Krey S, Steffee WP 1989 Exercise as an adjunct to weight loss and maintenance in moderately obese subjects. American Journal of Clinical Nutrition 49:1115–1123.

Powell KE, Thompson PD, Coopersen CJ, Kendrick JS 1987 Physical activity and the incidence of coronary heart disease Annual Review of Public Health 8:253–287.

Prentice AM, Jebb SA 1995 Obesity in Britain: gluttony or sloth? BMJ 311:437–439

Prochaska JO, DiClemente CC 1986 The transtheoretical approach. In: Norcross JC (ed) Handbook of Eclectic Psychotherapy. Brunner Mazel, New York.

Saris WH 2001 Very-low-calorie diets and sustained weight loss. Obesity Research 9(suppl 4):295S–301S.

Tate DF, Wing RR, Winett RA 2001 Using internet technology to deliver a behavioral weight loss program. Journal of the American Medical Association 285(9):1172–1177.

Wadden TA 1993 Treatment of obesity by moderate and severe caloric restriction: results of clinical research trials. Annals of Internal Medicine 119:688–693.

Wannamethee SG, Shaper AG 2003 Alcohol, body weight and weight gain in middle-aged men. American Journal of Clinical Nutrition 77(5):1312–1317.

Wood PD, Stefanick ML, Williams PT, Haskell WL 1991 The effects on plasma lipoproteins of a prudent weight reducing diet, with or without exercise, in overweight men and women. New England Journal of Medicine 325(7): 461–466.

Chapter 7

James WPT, Astrup A, Finer N et al 2000 Effect of sibutramine on weight maintenance after weight loss: a randomised trial. Lancet 356: 2119-2125.

Sjostrom L et al 1998 Randomized placebo-controlled trial of Orlistat for weight loss and prevention of weight regain in obese patients. European Multicentre Orlistat Study Group. Lancet 352:167–172

Torgerson JS et al 2004 XENDOS. Diabetes Care 27(1):155–161

Chapter 8

Balsiger BM, Murr MM, Poggio JL, Sarr MG 2000 Bariatric surgery. Surgery for weight control in patients with morbid obesity. Medical Clinics of North America 84(2):477–489.

Chambers R et al 2000 Weight loss, weight maintenance and improved cardiac risk factors after 2 years of treatment with orlistat for obesity. Obesity Research 8:49–61

Chung F, Mezei G, Tong D 1999 Pre-existing medical conditions as predictors of adverse events in day-case surgery. British Journal of Anaesthiology 83:262–270.

Eichenberger A, Proietti S, Wicky S et al 2002 Morbid obesity and postoperative pulmonary atelectasis: an underestimated problem. Anesthesia and Analgesia 95(6):1788–1792.

Mason EE, Tang S, Renquiat KE, et al 1997 Decade of change in obesity surgery Obesity Surgery 7:189–197.

NICE (National Institute for Clinical Excellence) 2002 Technical appraisal No 46. Surgery to aid weight reduction for people with morbid obesity. NICE, London. Online. Available: www.nice.org.uk

Ogunnaike BO, Jones SB, Jones DB et al 2002 Anesthetic considerations for bariatric surgery. Anesthesia and Analgesia 95(6):1793–1805.

Chapter 9

Epstein LH et al 1987 Stability of food preferences during weight control. Behavior Modification 11:87–101

Epstein LH et al 1995 Effects of decreasing sedentary behaviour and increasing activity in weight change in obese children. Health Psychology 14:109–115

Prentice AM, Jebb SA 1995 Obesity in Britain: gluttony or sloth? BMJ 311:437–439

Sinha R et al 2002 Prevalence of impaired glucose tolerance among children and adolescents with marked obesity. New England Journal of Medicine 346(11):802–810

Sorof J, Daniels S 2002 Obesity hypertension in children: a problem of epidemic proportions. Hypertension 40(4):441–7.

Chapter 10

Jung RT 1997 Obesity as a disease. British Medical Bulletin 53(2):307-21.

Chapter 11

World Health Organization Obesity: preventing and managing the global epidemic. WHO Technical Report Series, No. 894. Geneva, World Health Organization. Online. Available: www.who.int/nut/publications.htm

World Health Organization Diet, nutrition and the prevention of chronic diseases. Report of a joint WHO/FAO expert consultation. WHO Technical Report Series, No. 916. Geneva, World Health Organization. Online. Available: www.who.int/nut/publications.htm

Chapter 12

Despres JP 2004 Rimonabant in obesity. American College Cardiology 53rd Annual Scientific Session: late-breaking clinical trials

Haslam DW 2000 Treating obesity. Family Medicine 4(2):25–28.

LIST OF PATIENT QUESTIONS

INDEX

Weight loss (*cont'd*)
    see also Physical activity
  physiological benefits, **43**
  'plateau' effect, 123
  pseudotumour cerebri treatment, 74
  rapid, gallstone risk, 60
  self-esteem improvement, 69
  sleep apnoea treatment, 63
  stroke risk reduced, 47
Weight management, 26
  access for all social groups, 81
  indications, 176
  men, 81
  'stages of change', **113,** 113–114
  successful, criteria in children, 166
  see also Management
Weight management clinics, 171–182,
    180
  appointment frequency, 178
  clinical investigations, 177
  equipment, 173
  goal setting, 174–175, 178
  ideal, features, 173
  issues to raise with patients, 174
  numbers attending, 176–177
  patient selection, 176–177, 197
  'readiness to change' *see* 'Readiness to
    change'
  referrals, 178
  self-help, 177–178
  during working hours, 81
Weight Watchers diet, 100–101
Western dietary habits, 9–10

Will power, 25–26
Women, obesity in, 35–39
  infertility, 36
  self-confidence effects, 67
  surgery contraindications, 147
World Health Organization (WHO)
  *Diet, nutrition and prevention of chronic
    diseases,* 105
  metabolic syndrome definition, 40
  obesity definition, 4

X

Xanthelasmata, 59
XENDOS trial, 53, 134–136, **135**
Xenical® *see* Orlistat
Xenical in the Prevention of Diabetes in
  Obese Subjects (XENDOS), 53,
  134–136, **135**

Y

Young women, self-confidence loss, 67
'Yo-yo' dieting, 60, 89

Z

Zone diet, 97
Zyban®, **186**
Zyprexa®, **130**